CONJUNCTIONS

Conjunctions engages separately and connectively with therapeutic social work practice, psychoanalytically informed research methods, and philosophy, as well as contemporary human service organizational cultures and predicaments and the societal dynamics affecting social work and psychoanalysis. The chapters are gathered into several thematic sections: Practice; Organizations; Politics, Policy, and Culture; Research; and a final chapter on death, dying, and social work.

The writing on each topic uses a blend of psychoanalysis, social theory, and philosophy to illuminate and develop a psycho-social account of individual, organizational, and social processes and dynamics. Andrew Cooper draws directly upon his own and others' lived experience of clinical work, organizational stresses and strains, social processes, and research to generate conceptualized accounts of inner and outer experiential worlds in the hope of mobilizing emotional and thinking responses in his readership. *Conjunctions* is therefore intended to be an intervention in modern professional, therapeutic and social life, as well as a contribution to understanding it.

Andrew Cooper, a registered social worker and psychoanalytic psychotherapist, is Professor of Social Work at the Tavistock Centre and the University of East London. He continues to practise as a clinical social worker in the Adolescent Family Therapy service at the Tavistock, leads the Professional Doctorate in Social Work and Social Care programmes there, and works as a consultant to teams and organizations. In addition to his book *Borderline Welfare: Fear and Fear of Feeling in Modern Welfare* (co-authored with J. Lousada, 2005), he has written widely about therapeutic and relationship-based social work practice and research as well as the policy contexts that support or impede these practices.

Tavistock Clinic Series

Margot Waddell, Jocelyn Catty, & Kate Stratton (Series Editors)

Recent titles in the Tavistock Clinic Series

Addictive States of Mind, *edited by Marion Bower, Rob Hale, & Heather Wood*
Assessment in Child Psychotherapy, *edited by Margaret Rustin and Emanuela Quagliata*
Childhood Depression: A Place for Psychotherapy, *edited by Judith Trowell, with Gillian Miles*
Consultations in Psychoanalytic Psychotherapy, *edited by R. Peter Hobson*
Contemporary Developments in Adult and Young Adult Therapy. The Work of the Tavistock and Portman Clinics, Vol. 1, *edited by Alessandra Lemma*
Couple Dynamics: Psychoanalytic Perspectives in Work with the Individual, the Couple, and the Group, *edited by Aleksandra Novakovic*
Doing Things Differently: The Influence of Donald Meltzer on Psychoanalytic Theory and Practice, *edited by Margaret Cohen & Alberto Hahn*
Inside Lives: Psychoanalysis and the Growth of the Personality, *by Margot Waddell*
Internal Landscapes and Foreign Bodies: Eating Disorders and Other Pathologies, *by Gianna Williams*
Living on the Border: Psychotic Processes in the Individual, the Couple, and the Group, *edited by David Bell & Aleksandra Novakovic*
Making Room for Madness in Mental Health: The Psychoanalytic Understanding of Psychotic Communication, *by Marcus Evans*
Melanie Klein Revisited: Pioneer and Revolutionary in the Psychoanalysis of Young Children, *by Susan Sherwin-White*
Oedipus and the Couple, *edited by Francis Grier*
Organization in the Mind: Psychoanalysis, Group Relations, and Organizational Consultancy, *by David Armstrong, edited by Robert French*
Psychoanalysis and Culture: A Kleinian Perspective, *edited by David Bell*
Reason and Passion: A Celebration of the Work of Hanna Segal, *edited by David Bell*
Short-Term Psychoanalytic Psychotherapy for Adolescents with Depression: A Treatment Manual, *edited by Jocelyn Catty*
Sibling Matters: A Psychoanalytic, Developmental, and Systemic Approach, *edited by Debbie Hindle & Susan Sherwin-White*
Social Defences against Anxiety: Explorations in a Paradigm, *edited by David Armstrong & Michael Rustin*
Surviving Space: Papers on Infant Observation, *edited by Andrew Briggs*
Talking Cure: Mind and Method of the Tavistock Clinic, *edited by David Taylor*
The Anorexic Mind, *by Marilyn Lawrence*
The Groups Book. Psychoanalytic Group Therapy: Principles and Practice, *edited by Caroline Garland*
Therapeutic Care for Refugees: No Place Like Home, *edited by Renos Papadopoulos*
Thinking Space: Promoting Thinking about Race, Culture, and Diversity in Psychotherapy and Beyond, *edited by Frank Lowe*
Towards Belonging: Negotiating New Relationships for Adopted Children and Those in Care, *edited by Andrew Briggs*
Turning the Tide: A Psychoanalytic Approach to Mental Illness. The Work of the Fitzjohn's Unit, *edited by Rael Meyerowitz & David Bell*
Understanding Trauma: A Psychoanalytic Approach, *edited by Caroline Garland*
Waiting to Be Found: Papers on Children in Care, *edited by Andrew Briggs*
"What Can the Matter Be?": Therapeutic Interventions with Parents, Infants, and Young Children, *edited by Louise Emanuel & Elizabeth Bradley*
Young Child Observation: A Development in the Theory and Method of Infant Observation, *edited by Simonetta M. G. Adamo & Margaret Rustin*

CONJUNCTIONS

Social Work, Psychoanalysis, and Society

Andrew Cooper

Routledge
Taylor & Francis Group
LONDON AND NEW YORK

First published 2018
by Routledge
2 Park Square, Milton Park, Abingdon, Oxon OX14 4RN

and by Routledge
52 Vanderbilt Avenue, New York, NY 10017

Routledge is an imprint of the Taylor & Francis Group, an informa business

British Library Cataloguing in Publication Data

A catalogue record for this book is available from the British Library

Edited, designed, and typeset in Optima and Palatino
by Communication Crafts, East Grinstead

Printed and bound by CPI Group (UK) Ltd, Croydon, CR0 4YY

For Daniel and Rachael

CONTENTS

SERIES EDITORS' PREFACE

Margot Waddell, Jocelyn Catty, & Kate Stratton

Since it was founded in 1920, the Tavistock Clinic—now the Tavistock and Portman NHS Foundation Trust—has developed a wide range of developmental approaches to mental health which have been strongly influenced by the ideas of psychoanalysis. It has also adopted systemic family therapy as a theoretical model and a clinical approach to family problems. The Tavistock is now one of the largest mental health training institutions in Britain. It teaches up to 600 students a year on postgraduate, doctoral, and qualifying courses in social work, systemic psychotherapy, psychology, psychiatry, nursing, and child, adolescent, and adult psychotherapy, along with 2,000 multidisciplinary clinicians, social workers, and teachers attending Continuing Professional Development courses and conferences on psychoanalytic observation, psychoanalytic thinking, and management and leadership in a range of clinical and community settings.

The Tavistock's philosophy aims at promoting therapeutic methods in mental health. Its work is based on the clinical expertise that is also the basis of its consultancy and research activities. The aim of this Series is to make available to the reading public the clinical, theoretical, and research work that is most influential at the Tavistock. The Series sets out new approaches in the understanding and treatment of psychological disturbance in children, adolescents, and adults, both as individuals and in families.

Conjunctions: Social Work, Psychoanalysis, and Society could not be a more fitting successor to the book that Andrew Cooper and his co-author Julian Lousada published in the early days of the Tavistock Clinic Series, *Borderline Welfare: Feeling and Fear of Feeling in Modern Welfare* (2005). The "conjunctions" lie both in the humanity with which Cooper, now as sole author, continues to explore challenging and uncomfortable realities, and in the coherence and vividness with which he brings them alive in the detail of the chapters. *Conjunctions* engages with the most deeply painful areas of social work practice—child protection, child abuse, and institutional racism, to mention but a few, are near the centre and are appropriately explored.

The introduction to the book expresses Cooper's notion of "conjunction" very precisely: "In Praise of Tragedy: Social Work, Psychoanalysis, and Society". The subsequent chapters convey Cooper's thinking in his chosen style of writing—what he himself describes as "fluid, exploratory, and associative". In one sense, the book describes the inside story of the choice of profession, a choice that is presented both in movingly personal terms—what it was about the author's background that led him towards social work itself—and, later, in the deeper meaning of social work as an activity and as one of carrying a wider social purpose. He describes the "choice" of social work, for him, as "a way of continuing to try to heal my whole family" and, quite rightly, comments that "death and dying are transgenerational processes. How the generations that preceded us handle them profoundly affects each one of us". And, as he so powerfully relates, he chose a profession that continually faces some of the hardest social and political challenges and conflicts that beleaguer so hard-pressed an area of public work. The book goes to the core of what some would call the current crisis in social work training and practice and in the systems of social care more generally.

Cooper speaks of the "pyrrhic victory" of politics over casework and what led to a collapse of confidence in social work training and practice of the kind that informed his own training many years ago. The following sums it up: "values without the means to enact them are largely empty. Equally, working methods without values to guide them are blind." As he points out, the obvious question of how actually to *do* social work seldom, in fact, finds its way to professional pages. In the well-documented situations of accusation and vilification, it is common to find the social worker as the "fall guy", the "scapegoat", when it is actually the system that fails those who throw their hat into the ring of trying to help with the fundamental inequalities of the human condition. Cooper's question is not one of how to eradicate cruelty, abuse, or deprivation but of how to limit, manage, contain, recognize, and understand them.

In this area, we encounter yet another "conjunction" that needs to be embedded somewhere in the work so movingly described by Cooper: the role of psychotherapy and of psychoanalytic thinking in the conduct of people's engagement with this intensely demanding, indeed scarcely manageable endeavour. Cooper himself trained as a psychotherapist and brought this way of thinking to his long-term post as Professor of Social Work at the Tavistock, where, for many years, he has worked as a "psycho-social thinker, researcher, and practitioner". He describes how the "line between my social work and psychotherapeutic identities became fuzzier, although I maintained a clear sense of the 'discipline' and boundaries required to practise effectively in different contexts". The complexities surrounding the professions of social work, of psychotherapy, and of psychoanalysis are beautifully laid out in relation to the historical sweep of these professions' development and the social and political crises in the current state of affairs.

Cooper's aim—one that he fulfils so impressively—is to "bring something alive for readers, as much as to transmit knowledge". This position brings with it a rare insight and a sensitivity of expression that can be hard to find in these ever more simplifying and polarizing times. The chapter titles are enticing and immediately draw the reader into Cooper's way of arguing and thinking: "The Shock of the Real" (chapter 9), "Containing Tensions" (chapter 10), "'Be Quiet and Listen'" (chapter 11). One way or another, such topics have long been, and continue to be, ones that describe the elusive notion of the "Tavistock Model"—across all disciplines—and constitute a rather powerful summation of the work described in the foregoing books in the Tavistock Clinic Series.

ACKNOWLEDGEMENTS

My first thanks are due to Margot Waddell, who has been a supportive and enthusiastic editor from the moment I met with her to propose this book. Jocelyn Catty and Rod Tweedy have been expert chaperones and containers during the later stages of author anxiety. The co-authors of the three originally jointly authored chapters and papers included here have all been generous in their agreement to let me re-publish amended versions of our texts. Thank you to Amanda Lees, Julian Lousada, and Bernadette Wren. My best thinking is undertaken in dialogue and collaboration with others, and they are just a few among the many whose influence is central to the writing that follows. My friends Tim Dartington, Julian Lousada, Harvey Taylor, John Pitts, Claudio Esposito and my friend and brother Ron have been a source of intellectual stimulation, excitement, encouragement, understanding, solace, and much more over the years. The Victoria Stakes played its part. Agnes Bryan, Clare Parkinson, Liz Webb, Gillian Ruch, Jane Herd, Anna Harvey, and Helen Hingley-Jones have been great colleagues, collaborators, and friends too. My friends Pru Chamberlayne, Tom Wengraf, Barry Richards, Jo Brown, Daniel Herron, and Gareth Price have all helped sustain and nourish me. Thanks also to Amrik for help with diagrams, to the staff at Routledge who managed the final stages of production and printing, and to Eric King who was a most responsive and attentive copyeditor.

I do not like referring to participants on the various training programmes at the Tavistock as "students", since most of them are more experienced and capable practitioners than me, and at least equally able thinkers. Likewise the various doctoral candidates whose work I have examined over the years. So my heartfelt thanks to the huge number of professional colleagues with whom I have been privileged to engage in learning and teaching over the years. A number of you feature in this book, and I am especially grateful to Laura Harris, Ekim Erdogan, Sylvia Smith, Katharine Scanlan, Raelton Gibbs, Nicola O'Sullivan, Stephen Jordan, Jude Deacon, Judy Foster, Kathleen Russell, Nina Ezekiel, Philippe Mandin, Anna Harvey, Denise Turner, and Amanda Lees.

The members of the Tavistock Policy Seminar steering group have all made their presence felt in this book. Our meetings have always been creative, spontaneous, surprising, and occasionally riotous and delinquent. The work of these seminars has been original and inspiring, and the ethos of this project is threaded through the chapters of the book.

Colleagues and friends in my "other organization", the Centre for Social Work Practice, have been a source of hope that it's possible to get stuff done without excess bureaucratic impediments, and we have achieved some good things together for social work and made a difference.

I have needed a lot of therapeutic help during my life, and the influence of a number of therapists, and of my own patients and supervisors, is a less visible presence in the book. It seems all right now to mention my training therapist, Margaret Arden, by name. She died a few years ago, but I hope that something of her true independence of mind and spirit is alive in the pages of the book.

My membership of the Tavistock Adolescent Department Family Therapy Service and workshop has been a rich and vital source of clinical development, creativity, and fulfilment, and I thank the many colleagues and families with whom it's been a privilege to work.

My biggest vote of thanks is to my family—to Heather for her enduring love and encouragement as well as her astute intellectual and academic engagement, and to my two extraordinary and beautiful children, Daniel and Rachael. The papers and chapters that comprise this book were mostly written during the astonishing years across which our family formed and grew. Creative intellectual work has many sources, and my truest debt is to them.

* * *

Earlier versions of the following chapters were originally published as listed below and are republished with amendments by permission of the respective publishers.

Chapter 1: A. Cooper, "The Use of Self in Social Work Practice", in M. Bower & R. Solomon (Eds.), *What Social Workers Need to Know: A Psychoanalytic Approach* (London: Routledge, 2017), pp. 109–123.

Chapter 2: A. Cooper, "Emotional and Relational Capacities for Doing Child Protection Work", in L. Waterhouse & J. McGhee (Eds.), *Challenging Child Protection* (London: Jessica Kingsley, 2015), pp. 141–153.

Chapter 3: A. Cooper, "Legend, Myth and Idea: On the Fate of a Great Paper", *British Journal of Psychotherapy*, 26 (No. 2, 2010): 219–227.

Chapter 4: A. Cooper & A. Lees, "Spotlit: Defences against Anxiety in Contemporary Human Service Organizations", in D. Armstrong & M. Rustin (Eds.), *Social Defences against Anxiety: Explorations in the Paradigm* (London: Karnac, 2014), pp. 239–255.

Chapter 5: A. Cooper, "Talk Talk: Theories and Practices for Turbulent Times", in A. Lemma (Ed.), *Contemporary Developments in Adult and Young Adult Therapy: The Work of the Tavistock and Portman Clinics* (London: Karnac, 2012), pp. 19–41.

Chapter 6: A. Cooper, "Institutional Racism: Can Psychotherapy Change?", *British Journal of Psychotherapy, 26* (No. 4, 2010): 486–501.

Chapter 8: A. Cooper, "A Short Psychosocial History of British Child Abuse and Protection: Case Studies in Problems of Mourning in the Public Sphere", *Journal of Social Work Practice, 28* (No. 3, 2014): 271–285.

Chapter 9: A. Cooper & J. Lousada, "The Shock of the Real: Psychoanalysis, Modernity, Survival", in A. Lemma & M. Patrick (Eds.), *Off the Couch: Contemporary Psychoanalytic Applications* (London: Routledge, 2010), pp. 33–45.

Chapter 10: A. Cooper, "Containing Tensions: Psychoanalysis and Modern Policymaking", *Juncture, 22* (No. 2, 2015): 157–163.

Chapter 11: A. Cooper, "Be Quiet and Listen: Emotion, Public Policy and Social Totality", in S. Day Sclater, D. W. Jones, H. Price, & C. Yates (Eds.), *Emotion: New Psychosocial Perspectives* (London: Routledge, 2009), pp. 169–182.

Chapter 12: A. Cooper, "Hearing the Grass Grow: Emotional and Epistemological Challenges of Practice Near Research", *Journal of Social Work Practice, 23* (No. 4, 2009): 429–442.

Chapter 13: A. Cooper & B. Wren, "Front-Line Services, Complexity, Research and Policy", *Psychoanalytic Psychotherapy, 26* (No. 3, 2012): 199–210.

Chapter 15: A. Cooper, "Soft Eyes: Observation as Research", in H. Hingley-Jones, C. Parkinson, & L. Allain (Eds.), *Observation in Health and Social Care* (London: Jessica Kingsley, 2017), pp. 177–199.

CONJUNCTIONS

Introduction

In praise of tragedy: social work, psychoanalysis, and society

Writing differently

Sometime in the mid-1990s my approach to writing professional and academic papers and communications changed. I relaxed my tendency to produce tightly structured, rigorously analytical and evidenced scripts conforming to traditional academic conventions of argumentation in favour of a more fluid, exploratory, and associative style of writing. I can recall the moment when I realized I was allowing this to happen. The experience was both exhilarating and rather frightening. I would set out to write with no clear idea of what would emerge and just follow where my trains of thought led me. Inevitably, the first products of this experiment were rather shapeless and opaque. Gradually, I learned to reintroduce communicative form, academic coherence, and clarity of intellectual purpose into the writing, but always now as a second-order preoccupation. The idea of "being led by my trains of thought", rather than applying a formalized logic to the topic, became key.

Some years earlier, in a seminar on Freud's papers on technique, one of my teachers had observed that the ability to genuinely "free associate" is something that normally "arrives" for the patient towards the end of a psychoanalytic therapy, rather than being the methodological premise on which the process of psychotherapy rests. This was my experience. The capacity to "freely associate" was an achievement, a discovery, a developmental milestone, a recovery of spontaneity and playfulness which undid what I now saw as a more defensive apparatus of conventional intellectual rigour. The consequences of this for my career as a writer, scholar, and researcher were profound. Writing became a creative act, as much a performative intervention as an attempt to extend a body of knowledge, and I believe I found my own distinctive "voice". The downside was that my scholarly products became rather idiosyncratic and hard to categorize, a problem in relation to the emerging culture of metrics in academic performance assessments.

In the ensuing years, I have had a clear sense that some people respond warmly and enthusiastically to this way of writing, while others may be unsettled, bemused, and possibly rather disdainful of my lack of what they see as academic rigour. For myself, there was no going back. But I too have sometimes wondered whether this mode of production was not just an excuse for a degree of intellectual laziness, especially when I sensed my communications assuming a polemical or even moralizing tone. There is a very serious point to the rigours and disciplines of reasoned argumentation in the Western liberal academy, but equally these can, and often do, act as a constraining framework, extruding passion and vital sources of authorial lived experience in favour of a normatively driven intellectual production process organized by excess rationality.

Conjunctions

There are traceable connections between the personal "paradigm" of knowledge generation I forged, social work, the practice and experience of psychoanalytic therapy, and the contemporary intellectual landscape. I first encountered "psycho-social studies" in 1995 when I became external examiner for the degree programme of the same name at the University of East London. PSS, as it is generally now known, subsequently flourished and developed in a number of universities around the UK. Rooted in a creative interplay between modern sociology and various forms of psychoanalytic practice and theory, it encourages and supports a fluid, creative, and dynamic approach to research, knowledge, and their relationship to practice in the "real world" that social workers and therapists, among others, are primarily engaged with. Increasingly, I identified myself as a psycho-social thinker, researcher, and practitioner, and the line between my social work and psychotherapeutic identities became fuzzier, although I maintained a clear sense of the "discipline" and boundaries required to practise effectively in different contexts. As Paul Hoggett has argued, "The hyphen in psycho-social signifies a difference that cannot be dissolved. It therefore opens up the space for thinking. . . . In Winnicott's (1971b, p. 103) words it connotes the link that both joins and separates, the place where things do not fit but should fit" (2008, p. 383).

There was a sense of "coming home" in all of this. The distant origins and first appearance of the term "psycho-social" are somewhat disputed, but for me they are clear. As a social worker in training in the early 1980s, I studied the early edition of Florence Hollis's classic text *Casework: A Psychosocial Therapy* (Wood & Hollis, 1990), a sophisticated model of practice that drew on American psychoanalysis and social work theory to create a coherent framework for how to work with "persons-in-situation". Not just a person or just a context, but both—and, crucially, the third entity that is produced by the conjunction of the first two. Social work and social workers "live" in these transitional zones, in the difficult spaces between people, between people and their adverse circumstances and histories, between inner and outer worlds of experience, between the realms of private troubles and public issues, between the individual and the family, between the state and civil society, between past, present, and future—the list of binary pairings that they must negotiate is endless. But perhaps the most central dilemma, upon the horns of which social work has often impaled itself, is between the imperative to engage with the here-and-now circumstances of the suffering individual, and the aspiration to fight for a more just and equal society that will ameliorate suffering in general.

At the time I entered social work, this tension had become a split that had developed into a civil war between psychoanalytic casework and "radical social work" that propounded a structuralist, anti-psychologistic, and activist stance for the profession. Casework was accused of reductionism, individualism, and victim blaming and generally demonized as all things reactionary. I never accepted this oppositional framing, and much of my career and writing has been devoted to conjoining a depth psychoanalytic understanding of our task with a commitment to political critique and the pursuit of increased social justice. An excellent concise articulation of a non-binary, integrated systems–psychodynamic conception of the social work enterprise has recently been published (Hingley-Jones & Ruch, 2016). This is one theme, or thread, that links the different chapters in this book, which were originally written across a twenty-year time span. I think there are several other threads that (I hope) bind the book into something more than just a volume of "collected papers".

The two tasks

First, there is a preoccupation with what exactly social work is, and what it exists to accomplish. At various points in the book I broach the idea that social work has at least two primary tasks in society. The overt task could be summarized as the protection and safeguarding of vulnerable children and adults, the amelioration of relationships and circumstances creating adversity and suffering in families, individuals, and communities, and intervening to support people in difficult and painful lifespan-related transitions. But there is a covert or "under-the-surface" primary task as well, which is about protecting wider society from too much exposure to the anxiety associated with the cruelty, neglect, murderousness, violence, and mental pain perpetrated by citizens upon one another, or just endured because of misfortune.

There are complex tensions between these two tasks. On the one hand, it seems appropriate that a profession functions as a "specialized work group" on behalf of the remainder of society, relieving it from worry about what may be happening "just down the street", as I put it at one point (see chapter 12). I sometimes liken social work to the job done by the sewage industry—quietly and effectively disposing of, detoxifying, recycling, and managing the vast and inevitable consequences of the ordinary human fact that each of us needs to piss and shit each day. We don't think much about the complex systems required to perform this social task, or about the people who do it on our behalf, unless something goes wrong and sewage starts to overflow into the streets or back up in our toilets.

On the other hand, I argue that exactly because social workers, uniquely, *know* about the suffering and social marginalization of a wide variety of hidden populations in our midst, they have an ethical duty to bring this to public and political attention, to advocate and agitate for both "recognition" of these populations as "part of us" and not invisible "others", and more humane and better resourced provision for them. Some distinctive "ways of knowing" about these matters which we have evolved on Tavistock social work research degree programmes are explored in chapters 12, 14, and 15. However, some of the most painful periods in our professional history have been triggered when there has been a rupture in our capacity to "contain" within our professional systems our knowledge of dangerous aspects of human functioning. A child dies in especially painful circumstances, the matter is reported in the courts, and suddenly questions are being asked in the national media. Primitive dynamics of scapegoating and blame are mobilized, and, unhappily, social work has repeatedly become the "fall guy" in a process of collective hand-washing and disownment of responsibility for the suffering, damage, and anxiety endured by so many and routinely addressed by social workers. These issues are explored in chapter 8. The process of returning the genie to the bottle usually has damaging consequences for social work's ability to perform its first task, when excess regulation, surveillance, and proceduralization is implemented as the solution. The consequences for the helping professions of this process have been a continuing preoccupation, and my latest attempt to think these through is found in chapter 4.

Very few commentators have engaged in any depth with the "psycho-social nature of social work" in society as understood here. The best examples include Preston-Shoot and Agass (1990) and Shoesmith (2016). It is not comfortable, or necessarily appealing to potential recruits to the profession, to connote the central task of social work as engaging with conflicts of various kinds, but I believe that this a core truth that we should not evade. Shoesmith's compelling psycho-social analysis of the events that unfolded following the death of "Baby P" in 2007 culminates in her identification of a "cultural trope"—a deeply rooted assumption or belief that when things "go wrong" in relation to children at risk, "it's got to be the social workers' fault". She traces the detailed interplay of historical, ideological, professional, and political determinants of this "belief" using psychoanalytic thinking to disclose the collective unconscious processes at work.

Conflict, projections, and professional self-esteem

I hated the internal divisions in social work I encountered at the start of my career which tore us apart and left us empty of direction. Subsequently I have been endlessly dismayed at our professional passivity and lack of collective fight in the face of repeated assaults upon our integrity. Understanding this rather passive state of being is, in my view, a complex matter.

From time to time I am asked to speak publicly to social work audiences with a subsidiary request that I be "inspirational" or with a reminder that the aim of the event is to "celebrate" the achievements of social work. Commands of this kind give me a sinking feeling in my stomach. I am not against celebrating or inspiring, not least because (despite my sometimes gloomy diagnosis of our condition) there is much health and vigour and success in our profession. But my feeling is that these invitations have a defensive basis. "Please, we are subjected so much to unfair criticism, misrepresentation, and public contempt, so don't visit any more negative thoughts upon us. Come and give us an hour or two off from ourselves." My feeling is that this state of mind precisely captures the central problem about professional confidence which I want to explore.

People who suffer from low self-esteem lack an internal sense of their own value, self-worth, competence, potency, and capacity to offer good things to other people. It is easy (and in some instances true) to attribute this condition to a state of deficit—I wasn't loved enough, I lost the person who loved me most, it would all be all right if only I could find someone to provide the love and care I crave, and so on. More than once I have been asked to provide social work audiences with something that "feeds" them, as though the condition to be treated was literally one of hunger or starvation.

Invariably a more complicated picture lies just beneath the surface of this kind of presentation in individuals, quite a few of whom I have seen regularly in my psychotherapy practice. The situation causing suffering for the person may well have been, to some degree, directly internalized from circumstances in which the child, and now the adult, did not feel that there was "enough to go round", or that there was not the right kind of emotional responsiveness in the environment. But usually this state of affairs has become internalized as a set of self-perpetuating *beliefs* that form the basis of a fragile *self*. "I cannot and won't ask for or expect care and love because my self is worthless." This belief system, and the behaviours that flow into and out of it, gives rise first to an excessive dependence on external sources of confirmation of the self's value, but also an excessive vulnerability to external signs that it may not be valued. Criticism, sleights, or perceived failures to positively affirm the self lead to acute collapses of self-esteem, confirming the fundamental correctness of the core belief.

Sometimes we find that this picture is complicated by a defensive manoeuvre in which the sense of internal depletion and hunger is mastered via the attribution of this weak, needy, and "inferior" state to others, while the self is bolstered with a false sense of grandiosity. Poor self-esteem is not just the absence of positive self-regard, but a dynamic structure in which an authentic sense of self-worth rooted in a realistic evaluation of achievements, capacities, and possibilities is constantly undercut either by an excessively depreciated self-image or by a vastly inflated one that is maintained by attributing weakness and deficit to others. Often there will be complex oscillations between the two. Anyone who questions this state of affairs is likely to be met with a rather paranoid reaction; a questioning attitude towards the state of mind is experienced either as yet further criticism of the already depleted self, or as an effort to dismantle the fragile structure of defensive grandiosity, hence exposing the helpless and weak core of the self. (Extended discussion of these ideas can be found in Holmes, 2002.)

How does this analogy help us understand professional social work? Collectively, it seems to me that social work consistently adopts a rather cowering, ashamed, and diffident stance towards itself and the rest of the world, rather than an arrogant or grandiose one. I suggest that the collective counterpart of the dynamic structure in individuals outlined above is this: social workers project "real" competence and worth onto other professions and professionals in the multi-professional network, thus confirming a sense of themselves as depleted or inferior. Psychologists, doctors, psychotherapists, even nurses(!) are all seen as possessing a more solid, scientifically based and thus more legitimate core to their professional identity. This "scientific" base is ambivalently viewed, seen on the one hand as representing a reductionist, positivist, and objectifying world view that does scant justice to the psycho-social complexity of service users' lived experiences, but on the other as functioning as a ticket into professional credibility. However, all "identities" are relational, with self-worth and value to a significant degree a function of positioning within a projective network that generates a hierarchy. Within professions, the same struggles are played out among sub-disciplines, between, for example, clinical and educational psychologists, or among the many medical specialities. The senior doctor quoted in chapter 5 of this book who confidently asserted the superior, "first among equals" status of psychiatry in the mental health multidisciplinary hierarchy is engaged in the game of projective struggle for position and inter-group dominance and subordination I am describing here.

There are, of course, "real-world" correlates for the inter-group psychological struggles I outline above. A doctor's training is longer, more securely grounded in pure and applied research, and more rigorously examined and tested than a social worker's. Clinical and educational psychologists must achieve a doctoral level of academic study to qualify. The intensity of a psychoanalytic psychotherapist's experience with twice or three times weekly training cases is not matched by anything we require of social workers. As Harold Searles (1975) once remarked, in every transference there is a grain of truth (or more than a grain of truth). But within a few months of qualifying, social workers come to know about realities that most of their colleagues remain protected from, and they face making decisions as acute, painful, complex, and life-changing as those of any heart surgeon or neurologist. Yet we remain, for the most part, a diffident, under-confident, and uncertain bunch in our dealings with the world beyond our own professional community.

The vulnerable core

A central and real vulnerability of our professional identity concerns our failure to have developed and consolidated a set of reliable methods for doing what we are supposed to do—"help people" in a wide range of complex, adverse, and frequently conflicted circumstances and states of mind. We did once have such a repertoire, and it was taught and practised on qualifying social work trainings up and down the land. Task-centred casework, psycho-social casework, problem-solving casework, systemic casework, and more were at the centre of the curriculum I followed as a student and later taught as a social work educator. But faith in "methods" was one of the victims of the civil war I alluded to above. The pyrrhic victory of politics over casework led to a collapse of confidence in the importance of training workers to engage in sustained helping relationships. "Values" and to a lesser extent "theory" became the cornerstone of professional identity that filled the vacuum left behind. My own long engagement with certain strands of the "value base" in social work is reflected in chapters 6 and 16, which address questions of racism and anti-racist practice and theory, and some clues to the biographical roots of this engagement are found in one of them. But values without the means to enact them are largely empty. Equally, working methods without values to guide them are blind. Thus, a core reason for our difficulty in sustaining confidence in ourselves, especially in relation to colleagues in other disciplines, is rooted in this "emptiness", this deficit at the heart of our identity.

This situation is changing for the better, but slowly and uncertainly. In no particular order, an increasing number of experienced and qualified social workers are now also trained as play therapists, systemic therapists, psychoanalytic therapists, and so on, but they retain their original professional identity. Some organizational commitment to reintegrating sophisticated practice skills has also been in evidence—for example, in the Hackney "Reclaiming Social Work" model (Goodman, Trowler,& Munro, 2011). But too often social work looks *outside* itself to find the resources to bolster its internal lack. This is better than struggling on without seeking help, but the crucial further step of taking authority for our own development, and rediscovering or forging anew a set of strong, distinctively "social work" practice methodologies, seems harder to achieve. Of the books published in recent years that do seek to engage more strongly with real-world practice methodology, a significant number originate with practitioners based in, or closely associated with, the Tavistock Centre. Bower (2005a), Bower and Solomon (2017), Foster (2016), Ruch, Turney, and Ward (2010), and Wilson et al. (2011) are prominent contributions. The last of these is a textbook, designed to be a comprehensive introduction for qualifying students. Remarkably, it seems to be the only "textbook" ever published in the UK primarily addressed to questions of how to *do* social work .

The tragic dimension

Yet none of the above really explains why social work is afflicted with the identity problems I have tried to describe. The story I find most convincing runs as follows and recalls the idea of the "two tasks" outlined above. Social work was born and raised in circumstances of social disharmony, conflict, antagonism, and struggle. This is our birthright, the hand we were dealt in life. The family script handed to us by the wider society, in the crucible of our birth, was this: you are to be the bridge between order and chaos, civilization and anarchy, cruelty and tolerance, madness and sanity, moral integrity and perversion or depravity. Control your drunken father, rejuvenate your depressed mother, feed your hungry siblings, rehabilitate your villainous uncle, and so on and so on. Help rid us of these evils and we will love you; fail in your task and you fail to protect the honour of the family name, so we will vilify you. We know of these tribulations in our midst, and, while they trouble us greatly, we would rather not have to know too much, and it is your job to do what you can to protect us from knowing.

The everyday manifestations of these disharmonies and antagonisms become our caseloads. But pretty well all the varieties of suffering, misfortune, conflict, anxiety that we deal with have social and structural origins as well as psychological ones. We now know that in more equal societies there is just less mental illness, violent crime, depression, and child maltreatment (Wilkinson & Pickett, 2009). But in the most egalitarian, socially cohesive, democratic societies we have managed to create, plenty of all this is still going on. So, we must lay to rest a disabling myth once and for all. There are no utopias. The stuff that social workers deal with is part of the human condition, and always will be—just as inequalities will always be with us. The idea that human groups and societies are endowed with a fundamental essence that is harmonious and cooperative, distorted only by the competitive and destructive tendencies of capitalism or fascism, which if defeated would disclose the underlying purity of social being, is another formulation of this myth. As a colleague of mine who is an organizational consultant expresses it, "Institutions are abusive—families, communities, health services, care homes, churches, you name it, they all manifest abuse and cruelty—so the question is not how can we eradicate 'abuse', but how do we best equip ourselves to expect it, recognize it, understand its nature and then respond to contain and limit it?" This could seem like a counsel of despair, but surely it is just realism? A single example from experience may help to illuminate the importance of this stance.

A research student whose work I supervised used close observational methods to study the functioning of multi-professional network meetings in a family treatment service. The meetings are convened outside the judicial process but with respect to families who have been referred for assessment by the court (Mandin, 2014). Their goal is to create a more neutral "space" in which the many tensions of perspective surrounding and involving the family can be aired and if possible relaxed, allowing the family themselves a better chance of finding room to breathe in the assessment process. Families attend these meetings. One thing the observational stance has allowed this researcher to access more directly is the intensity, pain, and anxiety sitting at the heart of the whole process. One case involved a young mother who speaks no English with a 6-week-old baby and a father with a diagnosis of schizophrenia who has in the past attempted murder. If one just sits with this knowledge for a moment or two, the overwhelming power of the existential anxieties everyone is engaged with should become emotionally apparent. At a stark minimum, some possibilities are: child murder, adult murder, tiny baby separated for ever from mother, mother separated for ever from tiny baby, breakdown of marriage, adult mental breakdown. One or more of these is a probable, and certainly a feared, outcome of the eventual decision of the court, a decision that most of those present, family members included, are charged with influencing. Perhaps all these dreadful possibilities can be avoided, but, at this point in time, who knows? And how much uncertainty can we afford to bear?

Of course, it is not hard to guess that the observable behaviour, interactions, and emotional engagements of the many professionals in attendance at these meetings frequently seemed to this researcher to be displaced away from these facts and anxieties. There are sophisticated and useful theories to explain or interpret the way professionals relate, or don't relate, to one another under such conditions. But most of these theories do not really consider the significance of the core emotional experience I have tried to evoke. The elements of this experience are those of classical and modern tragic drama—Sophocles, Shakespeare, Arthur Miller. Terrible events unfold in these dramas, although there is usually a redemptive and hopeful strand to the narrative.

The profession of social work is one attempt by modern societies to *intervene* in our tragic narratives, rather than just "mentalize" them through cultural media such as theatre or film. We deploy the typically modern resources of social, psychological, and organizational theory in this project, and so we should. These are progressive and hopeful resources. But it is clear that they have not yet, and probably never will, conquer the tragic dimension.

Perhaps, then, it becomes a bit clearer what I believe are the core constituents of an adequate *theory* of social work, one that might help all its practitioners as well as the rest of society gain a more realistic and truthful perspective on its core *function*. In emphasizing this "tragic" dimension, I do not mean to recommend passivity or complacency, an attitude of acquiescence to fate. This is what a "tragic view of life" is sometimes wrongly interpreted to mean. Tragic drama surely always was an effort at "learning from experience", at achieving some better mastery of complex human predicaments and dilemmas. Our rationalist repertoire of risk-assessment protocols, checklists, manuals of procedure, interspersed with the odd case study, are perhaps the same fundamental project—just less interesting to read—and quite possibly no more effective.

The story of social work in Britain over the last thirty to forty years is not, in my view, a particularly happy or auspicious one. It certainly could have been better, and successive governments have indeed taken our profession as a soft target in their efforts to exert control over the professions generally. And yet personally I remain engaged, fascinated, fulfilled, and not at all ashamed by my professional identity as a social worker. I could describe my view of my own life in not dissimilar terms, if it comes to it. Stuff happened to me as quite a young man that probably could not have been prevented, which caused me considerable suffering and anxiety and altered the course of my life, including perhaps influencing me to become a social worker. Relationships, including a lot of professional relationship-based help, have for me been the single most important source of change, development, hope. and repair. Some of these biographical events are more fully narrated in chapter 16.

Sometimes, perhaps often, it is governments we need to stand up to, engage with robustly, fight with even. Social work is an arm of the state, in the same way the NHS is, but it needs to be more than that. Conventional policymaking processes have become very disconnected from people's lived experience, including the lived experiences of professionals. Policymakers in my experience occupy a kind of closed and emotionally sanitized world of assumptions, procedures, methods, and aims. Social workers, on the other hand, really *know* things about the lives of the marginalized, disadvantaged, the suffering, and the vulnerable. Chapters 10 and 11 explore the progressive possibilities of a policy culture grounded in the messy lived experience of people's lives. But we cannot expect ourselves as individuals, or others, to speak out alone. We really need the solidarity of strong organizations to support and protect us. To rediscover and reanimate our public and political identity would be to take up a less passive, more assertive, and therefore potentially more conflictual stance. Human development, whether individual, family, group, or societal, entails conflict and the working-through of conflict. These are central insights of both the psychoanalytic and the Marxist world views, which unashamedly underpin much of what is written in these pages.

And psychoanalysis?

As I write, Marxism has made a bit of a comeback on the British political stage, with the election of a Labour Party leader who seems more or less unafraid to refer his values and principles to this origin, and a president of the United States who is a direct threat to the advances made by liberal democracy. But who is listening to psychoanalysis in the modern era? Can psychoanalysis listen to its own many voices? Can it listen to the voices of others, especially less friendly ones? Returning from a holiday in France in August 2011, I was idly watching a TV screen in the airport departure lounge. Breaking news rippling past at the foot of the screen suddenly announced "Psychoanalyst Joyce

McDougall has died". In how many countries of the world would such an event be considered newsworthy, I wondered? This may not be the most scientific index of the global health or otherwise of psychoanalysis, but it is a place from which to start.

The contemporary survival agonies of the psychoanalytic community take numerous forms. Disentangling the interwoven strands of this distressed state is an important project, part of the work we must do in order to find a more secure place for psychoanalytic therapies in a changed and changing world. The task resembles, but of course cannot be the same as clinical psychoanalytic work itself. There is a rich, long, and diverse tradition of psychoanalytic thought and practice "off the couch" or "beyond the consulting room", originating with Freud himself. This is work that tries variously to illuminate the unconscious forces at work in group, organizational, social, and political processes and in the constitution of society itself. But the seemingly obvious reflexive move, in which psychoanalysis takes itself as its object and turns its unique form of "gaze" on its own social institutions, history, and cultural predicaments, is less common than it could be, or should be.

On the other hand, a debased and wild form of this potential for psychoanalytic self-understanding is all too familiar, one in which the inevitable and ordinary developmental struggles of a complex international professional community are degraded by "friendly fire", the cunning and often camouflaged decimation of colleagues with whom we have differences, using our own armoury of killer concepts—projection, splitting, rivalry, and so on—to characterize others' failings and betrayals. A few days after I began work at the Tavistock Clinic in 1996, I was drawn into conversation about a neighbouring institution, the Institute for Group Analysis, and what it represents. "Whatever they do, it's not psychoanalysis", I was informed. My interlocutor's tone suggested I would have no knowledge or opinions of my own on this subject, or, if I did, that I needed to be put straight as soon as possible. It was not a descriptive observation but a powerfully normative one, demarcating territory and positioning "them" as "not us". It was an act of closure, inhibiting curiosity, and, I felt, a subtle test of my fidelity to the institution I had recently joined—or at least to my colleague's preferred image of this institution.

The psychoanalytic community can no longer afford the dangers of such destructive self-absorption. As long as the rest of the world continued to give some sort of assent to psychoanalysis' own idea of its pre-eminence in the world of psychological therapy and theory, the self-harm inflicted by our collective narcissism was limited. All this has changed. For a hundred and twenty years or so, psychoanalysis was a huge success story and profoundly enriched a large part of humanity's view of itself. But now we are in a fight for survival. No one else cares about our internal disputes and schisms, or if they do it is merely to relish the manner in which they weaken us. To move beyond this state of affairs does not imply suppressing differences and debates, for these are indeed the motor of development and change. But we do require a combination of greater tolerance and increased humility about our place in the world. The two are linked. The narcissism of minor differences continually enacted within and among psychoanalytic communities reflects the arrogance with which we tend to disparage those poor creatures and traditions that lack the benefits of our wisdom. Arrogance, as Bion noted, is closely associated with stupidity, and in turn both may be reminders of a sense of underlying catastrophe. What might this be for psychoanalysis as a whole? These themes are examined more fully in chapters 5 and 9.

Interestingly, as with social work, I suggest that the answer lies in a profound sense of collective insecurity about identity and the basis of self-esteem. Psychoanalysis and psychotherapy have directly helped a small, mostly privileged section of the population. In Britain, wider access to publicly funded psychoanalytic work has declined from an already restricted base, which until the 1980s was mostly located in the traditions of psychiatric social work. It endured in a small number of NHS psychotherapy departments and therapeutic communities, but these are now being dismantled. This perilous state of affairs has been compounded by a deep reluctance to even seek admission to mainstream social and political structures such as professional regulation, which provide—albeit probably at the cost of certain necessary tensions and compromises—a significant degree of "social security".

With the notable exception of psychoanalytic child psychotherapy, which put down its first roots within the NHS, psychoanalysis and psychoanalytic psychotherapy are not proper professions in Britain (Taylor, 2013). Our institutions and individual members behave most of the time as though they are traditional professions and professionals, and both borrow extensively from the precepts and principles of mainstream professionalism. But this only serves to disguise the fact that our official social positioning is little different from that of astrologers, agony aunts, or acupuncturists. Our comparatively greater social authority derives from nineteenth- and twentieth-century cultural principles—an expectation that tradition, education, and professional integrity will elicit respect and trust, that "depth" engagement will ultimately find favour over "quick-fix" solutions—principles that can no longer bear the weight we require of them. In the context of a hierarchically ordered and stratified society, psychoanalysis successfully cultivated a certain kind of social transference to its own endeavours. But the glass frame that housed this delicate culture has cracked and broken, allowing a tangle of other therapeutic flowers and shrubs to spring up around us. In both domains, in social work and psychoanalysis, we need revised foundations for our continued legitimacy.

But this book is not a manifesto for the future. Before such a tract can be meaningfully written, there is more groundwork to do. To think the new thoughts that might be the well-springs of a different fertility, we first need to face unpalatable facts about ourselves, about the times in which we live, and about the imperfectability of our species. The root of this project is not so much intellectual as developmental, and this is the spirit in which this book is written.

That said, this introduction is not complete without a fulsome acknowledgement of the passionately central place that "the Tavistock" occupies in the chapters of this book. For very many of those who work there, the Tavi *has* got something "right" with its complex and sometimes internally fraught model of practice, education, and training and research. The Tavistock "model" is often referred to but rarely defined or codified. Chapter 5 is my attempt to set this right. Tavistock social work practice and thinking is a dimension of the much more complex whole that is the wider enterprise of the institution, and indeed its sibling organizations that bear the same name. The Tavistock has been at the heart of my professional life for more than two decades, but especially the project of developing and disseminating the work of the social work discipline. It has changed me irrevocably, entered my emotional and mental bloodstream, sustained me and rewarded me hugely—even if it has often maddened me too. Whatever, its influence can be heard in every chapter, sometimes as the bass line, sometimes as the melody, and frequently as the entire composition.

But tragedy of a different hue to the one evoked above also stalks the corridors of the Tavistock Centre and its satellites. The chapter dedicated to articulating the Tavistock "model" was originally written a few years ago, and since then the forces of managerialism, "modernization", and the pressures of market forces and austerity have made deep inroads into the solidaristic institutional culture that has sustained its work for nearly a century. Solidarity and collectivism of any kind are anathema to those who put their faith in the market and in an indiscriminate, corporate-dominated idea of "globalization". Such trajectories of tragedy need to be resisted and opposed. Of course this is easier said than achieved, and while antagonistic forces hold sway, the task is also to adapt and survive, an observation that resonates with the binocular concept of social work discussed above. Adaptation in the service of conserving good things in adverse conditions is sometimes the radical option. It doesn't make for a pure kind of political activism, but the alternative is unthinkable. I hope that this book is a contribution to both preserving and advancing the practices, ideas, and values that constitute the Tavistock project.

PART I

PRACTICE

CHAPTER ONE

The use of self in social work practice

Introduction

Relationship-based and therapeutic social work practice relies on us "using ourselves" as a resource in direct work with service users. But what do we mean by the "self" in this context, and how do we "use" it? In this chapter I explore some psychoanalytically based answers to these questions and present a number of case studies and clinical vignettes that illustrate different aspects of the use of self.

Effective therapeutic social work is not primarily about using theory to understand other people or ourselves. Rather, it concerns a capacity for attunement to our emotional experience of ourselves in relation to others, an attunement to the flow of emotional transactions between ourselves and our service users and colleagues which are occurring constantly whether we choose to recognize them or not. This is why the use of self is so important. Concepts like transference, countertransference, projection, and splitting can seem daunting, but they describe powerful processes that will destabilize our best intentions to practise effectively if we cannot track them and work with them as they are occurring. Equally, understanding how to recognize, track, and make sense of the emotional dynamics that are always alive in our work deepens our practice, improves our performance and our effectiveness and decision making, and helps protect us from the sometimes psychologically damaging impact of the work we do. In other words it is a core professional skill, perhaps *the* most central skill we need to develop, sustain, and hone.

The chapter begins with a detailed case study of one-to-one work and a series of reflective commentaries on this unfolding story. It then offers a further case study of multi-agency practice with a family where a new-born baby is deemed to be at risk, and some further reflective commentary. Finally, some brief extracts from a case and how it ended are presented. Along the way, a number of key concepts are introduced, and readers interested in pursuing the more theoretical aspects of the chapter can follow up the references provided. In particular, Marion Bower (2005a) has written a very helpful, concise introduction to key concepts. But the focus of the present chapter is on the immediacy and power of the "lived experience" of practice encounters, making sense of these, and the meaning of "using yourself" as a resource in the work.

A panic attack

A social worker in a voluntary-sector mental health organization began work with a socially isolated single man in his fifties. Mr A had been referred by his GP, who felt concerned about him but unable to clearly "diagnose" his problem. The GP described the man as "difficult" and complaining. He attended the practice frequently with relatively minor medical "complaints"—gastric symptoms, eye infections, and chest pains that did not respond to routine medication and for which tests could find no obvious cause.

The worker agreed a contract of sessions with Mr A, who accepted the offer but seemed noticeably reserved and perhaps rather cynical and suspicious of whether "it would do any good". After three meetings the worker felt he did know more *about* Mr A, but did not feel he had *got to know him* at all. Mr A expressed much disappointment with his life. He had hoped to be married and have children, and he felt his career had never taken off. He spoke of an older brother who had made his childhood miserable with teasing and bullying that his parents had never protected him from, and of a few friends, but the worker felt that these relationships were all very "thin". The worker tried to be empathic with Mr A's account of his life, but these efforts to make emotional contact with him were often met with a critical response. Mr A implied that the worker had misheard him and "got it wrong". At the start of each session following the first meeting, Mr A would refer to something the worker had said the previous week and again convey his dislike and disagreement. However, the worker did not completely recognize the remarks Mr A reported him having made. It was as though they had become "twisted" in some way, and it was this distorted version to which Mr A then reacted critically.

The main feeling the worker had was the sense of Mr A's isolation and loneliness, but he felt that the sessions had not led to any proper emotional contact with the sad or emotionally isolated aspect of his client. The worker found it hard to like Mr A and began to rather dread seeing him, feeling apprehensive about receiving yet more subtle criticism and confusing communications.

Then, during the fourth session, which on the face of it developed much as the previous ones had, the worker was gradually overtaken by an anxiety that Mr A might be suicidal. He could not really account for where this feeling came from, but it gripped him increasingly as the session progressed. Not feeling he had a real alliance with Mr A, and unsure about whether the feelings and thoughts were meaningful, he said nothing. But after the session, the worker became more and more anxious and panicky. What if Mr A attempted suicide and he had done nothing? Were his case notes written up fully? Should he be alerting the GP, but, if so, on what grounds? The state he found himself in did not feel like his usual professional self, which he believed to be normally quite composed. The worker realized that he could not really "think straight" and that something unusual had taken place, which he did not understand. He sought out his supervisor. He was fortunate to have access to a supervisor who was skilled in relationship-based work. What happens if you are not so fortunate is a question I take up later in the chapter.

The supervisor listened carefully and then made some suggestions. It seemed the worker had been "invaded" by these powerful feelings and anxieties during the session with Mr A. It did not feel convincing that this was actually the worker's "stuff", but more that he had been "taken over" by feelings that were definitely not his. Surely there might be reason to suppose that they did have some meaningful connection to his client? He fully acknowledged the worker's sense that he did not feel he had been able to "make contact" with Mr A at any deeper level and that, in turn, Mr A seemed to feel systematically misunderstood by the worker. So was it possible that these very powerful feelings were another form of communication and should be taken seriously?

Rather than feel too panicked, the worker might think that he now *had* made some contact with Mr A, or rather that Mr A had "got through" to him with his deeper anxieties—it just hadn't happened in words, or in the way the worker expected or hoped for.

The worker felt more settled, and his supervisor suggested that he needed to test out these hunches directly with Mr A at the next session. He helped the worker to think about ways to do this, at an appropriate moment in the flow of the session. So when he next met Mr A, the worker found an opportunity to say, "Now I have been able to get to know you a little, I have the sense that you often feel very lonely and isolated, and very disappointed with the way things have worked out in your life. I wonder whether at times you may feel really despairing, and perhaps have thoughts of suicide?" The impact of this remark on Mr A was definite, although quite subtle. He visibly relaxed slightly, looked hard at the worker, and said simply "Yes".

Reflecting on the process

What can we notice and learn from this account of the work with Mr A?

Engaging and creating the frame

First, it takes time to establish a working alliance with any service user, or family. Both parties are anxious and the early meetings will be full of uncertainty, as everyone works through their worries about whether they feel they can "work with this person". Salzberger-Wittenberg's (1970) beautifully simple and direct account of the way these anxieties are active for both worker and service user is a valuable resource that unpacks the fuller meaning of a statement by the psychoanalyst Wilfred Bion: "In every consulting room there ought to be two rather frightened people: the patient and the psycho-analyst. If they are not, one wonders why they are bothering to find out what everyone knows" (Bion, 1990, p. 5).

Second, while these early phases of the contact are being negotiated, the worker's most important role is simply to carry on being reliably "there". A consistent "frame" for the work, a regular appointment time and place, helps immeasurably, as well as an absolute commitment from the worker to honour these arrangements. Failing, suddenly changing, or being late for appointments will convey that the worker's mind is not really on the client and likely confirm worries in the service user that they are not worth the bother, that the worker cannot tolerate whatever difficulties the service user is carrying, and so on.

Recognizing and engaging with the transference

Third, the phenomenon we call the "transference", and its companion, the "countertransference", takes time to make itself known fully and clearly. In the case of Mr A, as in every case, there are early signs and signals, and we try to take notice of these and make sense of them. The worker very quickly has an experience that Mr A is not easy to get to know and is unable to present his problems in an open and clear way so that the two of them can "get down to work" on some issues. Perhaps, then, we gain some insight into why the GP made the referral—nothing the GP offered or provided or recommended seemed to work to make things better, and in the early sessions this is the social worker's experience as well. Service users who frustrate and perhaps make experienced staff feel deskilled are often handed over to another service. The hope is often as much that another agency will relieve the first one of the strain, anxiety, frustration, and guilt associated with a lack of progress than a genuine wish that the service user might be better helped. The referral itself may be freighted with such transferential material, and our recognition of this helps us orientate to the case we are taking on.

When a transference communication does leap to the fore, it often does so from "left field", catching us unaware and throwing us off balance. This is the nature of the "unconscious". If the state of mind causing anxiety for the client were better known and understood by them and hence communicable in words, it would all be much easier for us to understand and get to grips with. But painful or frightening unconscious processes are shaped and constrained by the defences the client has evolved to manage them. The worker needs to be emotionally available to receive both the defensive manifestations (often but not always hostile or rejecting) of the troubling mind states, as well as the communication of anxiety, panic, despair, or mental conflict that underlies the defences. In Mr A's case it seems the underlying feelings are of extreme loneliness, a fear or belief that he cannot be "reached" emotionally or that it will be painful and humiliating if he allows this. So he rejects efforts to reach him and seems to make the worker feel useless, hopeless, and angry. The latter "defensive" states of mind are what the worker first receives, but later he succeeds in making some tentative contact with other layers of Mr A's mind and feeling states.

Projective identification

In the case described here, the hypothesis is that the worker's "anxiety attack" is meaningful in a special sense, if only we can discover the meaning. It is the product of a powerful form of communication we call projective identification, in which one person succeeds in exporting a state of mind more or less directly "into" someone else who then comes to experience this state of mind as his own while simultaneously being aware that something has ambushed him internally. Casement's (1985) characterization of projective identification as "communication through impact" is a very helpful and accessible discussion of this process. In the case study, the worker experiences a tumult of disturbing thoughts, feelings, and confusion. He has the insight to suspect that something has "got into him" or under his psychological skin. But what, and how, and can he be sure? We might notice that in the midst of this experience he says he cannot "think straight", and be reminded of how he had noticed Mr A seeming to "twist" the worker's communications and feed them back to him. The worker's experience is that he is not "himself". This captures what being subject to an experience of projective identification is like. It is more powerful, direct, and perturbing to the worker than simple projection, in which one person may attribute qualities to another in a more explicit and symbolized form, although such processes occur on a subtle spectrum of intensity (Goretti, 2007).

Containment and using the "self" to make a difference

Once the worker has explored his experiences with the supervisor, who offers a suggestion about how to use them in the next session, the question becomes one of finding the confidence to do this. Psychoanalytic work has often been critiqued on the grounds that the worker or therapist may seem to take up a position of secretly and arrogantly "knowing the patient" better than the patient knows him/herself, or of laying claim to some "magical" type of understanding. The reality for any thoughtful practitioner is very different. We are groping in the dark much of the time, doing our best to think about the service user and to find a way to use our experiences to increase emotional contact with the deeper layers of anxiety and distress in our clients. Any interpretation of the service user's difficulties is always provisional and tentative and, most importantly, must be tested with them in a careful and sensitive manner. If an interpretation seems to "hit the spot", make the patient feel understood, and increase genuine emotional contact, then we can be more confident we are on a helpful track.

Mr A's response does seem to indicate that the formulation developed by worker and supervisor is accurate. However, it is useful to review and notice everything that has led up to this point. The worker's emotional receptivity is a key foundation. He is able to receive Mr A's critical and suspicious communications without rejection or retaliation; he tolerates the experience of becoming invaded by anxiety in the fourth session, and then his subsequent panicky state of mind; he uses his supervisor to "think with" in an open way; and out of this process, which unfolds over several weeks, some words take shape that, when sensitively delivered, appear to calm the service user and reach a deeper level of distress and fear within him. This process exemplifies the psychoanalytic idea of "containment" (Bion, 1962). It is both simple and yet subtle and complex. The steps involved in the containment process are first emotional receptivity, then tolerance of the suffering and confusion that ensues, and then an effort to think and make sense of these experiences, and finally "returning" the experiences to their originator in a new form that the person finds "digestible", meaningful, and helpful. We believe that this process replicates or re-enacts something of what goes on between a baby and its mother or primary caretaker in the period before the infant has the ability use words or even symbols to help make sense of its experiences, and when projective identification (see above) is the main means by which emotional distress is communicated to the mother.

Seeking help

The worker does the sensible thing and seeks help from his supervisor. His supervisor's response is thoughtful, neutral, and attentive in the service of making sense of professional experience. Unfortunately the quality and availability of supervisory or consultative help evoked here is in too short supply in contemporary social work agencies. But it is a vital element in the total picture involved in the "use of self" in practice. The fact is we cannot do this work alone, although with experience and the right training we become better able to manage complex and difficult practice encounters without seeking help all the time. A worker who can use his psychological experiences effectively will not to be ashamed or afraid of asking for help, of "not knowing" what is going on, or of feeling incompetent and confused. As we shall see a bit later in this chapter, struggling on with experiences like the above one lodged somewhere inside us, but unprocessed, is ultimately harmful in at least two ways: we miss vital information about how to help service users with their difficulties, and we become psychologically burdened and deskilled ourselves.

Of course, as workers in busy, hard-pressed front-line services, we do have a lot of other people on our minds, and many anxieties of our own, but these matters are not the service user's problem. Even if we are lucky enough to have access to a sensitive supervisor or manager, it is unlikely that he or she is available "on demand". Living with the uncomfortable feelings and thoughts that practice encounters throw up until we can find access to a reflective supervisor or colleague is just part of the job. Colleagues can help, of course, and most offices are alive with conversations about workers' recent encounters. But just "discharging" difficult feelings and thoughts does not usually lead to better understanding of the *meaning* of it all. A better grip on what difficult practice encounters mean is the real goal, and, echoing the therapeutic helping process itself, this usually needs another thinking mind with which to work.

Thus, a key message of this chapter is that relationship-based practice is not something you can practice in isolation. The power of case dynamics requires *organizational* attention, in particular the provision of reflective supervision as a standard part of agency life. As suggested, however, in practice this is often not available, so what is to be done? This is really a topic for another chapter, but one line of thought which owes something to group-relations thinking is to say that, as professionals, we need to "take our own authority" in asking our organizations for what we believe we need in order to practise well. Modern social work managers are hard-pressed people, but we can expect them to listen to us in a thoughtful manner—just as our service users have the right to expect this of front-line staff.

Two recent research studies that examine in minute qualitative depth the experiences of front-line child protection workers show how they may become in effect "secondarily traumatized" because of the long-term impact upon them of particular cases that they found impossible to process or make sense of (Noyes, 2015; O'Sullivan, 2017). A classic text that also brings alive the experience of front-line social work practice in a statutory setting is Janet Mattinson and colleagues' *Mate and Stalemate* (Mattinson, Sinclair, Coussell, & Morley, 1979). This book was based on action research undertaken in a London social services department in the late 1970s, and while some aspects of the service context now seem dated, the processes illustrated are as recognizable as ever.

So, what is this "self"?

The above discussion might reassure readers that when we speak about the use of self in social work, we are not referring simply to "gut feelings" or even "intuition", although both these notions play a part in the bigger picture of the professional self I am advancing in this chapter. The self I am interested in here is more a process than a "thing". It concerns our ability to scan, monitor, reflect upon, make sense of, and put to work our awareness of occupying a total field of experience (Ogden, 1999) in what I hope to have conveyed is a sophisticated and above all thoughtful and reflective manner. This "field" is not just subjective, but inter-subjective, which means that we are attending to the continual impact of ourselves on others, and of them on us. These relationship impacts are active at the conscious, preconscious, and unconscious levels of our own and others' experience.

Our task as workers is to know ourselves well enough, so that we can disentangle the influence of others upon ourselves, and us upon them, and thus make sense of how their anxieties, conflicts, and distress are being communicated. This distinction is partly captured by the idea of distinguishing the "personal" countertransference (what we might be projecting into our own perception of a situation) from the service-user countertransference (our registration of what they might be projecting into us). Personal psychotherapy is the most helpful way a worker can evolve the deeper capacities for "knowing themselves" that I am speaking of here. But there are other routes to deeper self-awareness, including some that reach parts of the self that individual therapy does not. Undertaking an experiential group relations event in which a large body of people come together, with a staff group of facilitators, for the sole purpose of studying their own behaviour and experiences in groups and inter-group processes, are one such route. The experience of undertaking an infant or young child observation, or of being a member of a "work-discussion group", are others. These experiences are not psychotherapy but, especially in combination, their impact on the development of the worker may be very similar.

However, good social work, and sound decision making cannot rely solely on the use of self as it is conceptualized here. We need our more cognitively oriented rational analytic faculties too in order to make sound assessments, decisions, and plans. Knowledge of child development theory and research and of organizational theory is crucial, and appropriate—though not unquestioning—respect for agency procedures is vital. There is a helpful discussion of the important balance to be struck between "intuition" and "reasoning" in Eileen Munro's work, including her reports into the state of the child protection system (Munro, 2010).

At the sharp end

How can we use the self in pressurized, multidisciplinary, front-line service contexts, when the opportunity to create a stable frame may be compromised and urgency, risk, and unexpected demands may undermine our best efforts to plan the work carefully? In a performance-driven and risk-averse practice culture, can therapeutic social work really still find a foothold? The answer is definitely "yes", but few writers have really tackled this. Heather Bailey's (2015) paper is an excellent account of how a worker can make huge advances in understanding a complex case through thoughtful reflection and follow though of an urgent, unplanned, and rather crisis-laden phone call. The "crisis" led Bailey to re-evaluate the kind of provision a traumatized child might need in order to feel contained and be able to develop.

In another paper about the Victoria Climbié report (Cooper, 2005b) I focused some attention on one passage from the mass of evidence and analysis presented. It concerns the evidence given by a senior social worker, which is first quoted, followed by some commentary of my own:

> "The third strategy meeting recommendation to seek some proof that the child was Kouao's, arose from a feeling she had when Kouao came into the office on 2 November that something was amiss in the interaction and bonding between Kouao and Victoria" (Laming, 2003, p. 179). Later this worker is directly quoted. "Part of me, with the feelings I got from the visit with mum, it must have been still something that was niggling at me and I suggested just to be on the safe side, just to be certain, just to make sure, that she was not returned to Manning's" (Laming, 2003, p. 187).
>
> The reason these short passages spring out is that they demonstrate, in the context of the report, a rare quality of emotional aliveness to the situation facing the worker. Something troubling and perturbing is registered and is being thought about. This speaks to what it means to have and make use of a professional relationship

> in child protection work. Through an emotionally alive relationship with the family, it is possible to access something of the nature of *their relationships*. In registering a sense of disturbance, a practitioner registers signs of the potential risks, dangers and disturbances in the family relationships. Such experiences are not sufficient grounds on which to act, of course, but they are necessary information that when ignored or reasoned away may be the first step on a path to tragedy. [Cooper, 2005b, p. 159]

Here we see an illustration of how crucially important it can be for a worker to trust her feelings, even if she cannot articulate their meaning very coherently. This case eventually ended in tragedy, of course, but without doubt the social worker quoted here made the right decision at the point in time she had the opportunity.

A baby at risk? A worker keeps her head . . .

A social worker in a busy children's services referral and assessment team was "collared" rather anxiously and urgently by her manager as she came in to work. A referral had been made by the local hospital maternity unit who were concerned about the parental care of a new-born baby boy with Downs syndrome. The main worry seemed to be the baby's father, who was described as extremely angry, blaming of the hospital staff for somehow causing his son's condition, and unable to relate to or hold the child. The baby's mother was also causing some concern. She had shown signs of bonding with her newborn, but she was also distracted and had failed one opportunity to visit her baby who was still in hospital.

The manager asked the worker to make an urgent visit to the family home to meet the parents and their 2-year-old daughter and then attend a professionals meeting at the hospital. On the basis of the hospital team's experience of the "aggressive" father, she advised strongly that the worker be accompanied on the home visit by a male social worker "to protect her from violence". Here, once again, we see that powerful feelings and anxieties are embedded within the referral process. The worker writes:

> However, I was concerned that an image of this family was being presented to me before I had even had any opportunity to connect with them. I was being invited to be fearful and defensive before I had even met the family, as if a state of mind that may have belonged to the hospital staff was being projected into me.

> I decided to make contact with the father before the arranged visit because I felt that if effective work was to take place with this family, an atmosphere of fear and anger needed to be avoided as much as possible. When I phoned father and spoke to him, my impression was of a man who certainly was angry but also expressed a lot of vulnerability. In my countertransference I did not feel afraid of this man, but concerned for what the family including the mother and the two-year-old were going through with this major life-changing trauma.
>
> I think with hindsight this initial phone call, and the feelings that I got from it that contrasted with the feelings I was being invited to have by the hospital professionals, was crucial in developing an effective therapeutic relationship with this family. It was as though I was able to then treat them as a family suffering as opposed to a family on the attack, and they were more able to welcome me in to the family as a potentially helpful figure.[1]

At the meeting with the family, the father remained angry and blaming of the NHS and the system. It emerged that the mother had never been offered, or maybe had not taken up, the chance of a second routine test to establish whether the foetus was healthy or not (the first test had been negative). Language difficulties may have played a role in this oversight.

> After introducing myself, father asked if I knew what had happened. By this it became clear that what he meant was how the hospital had let him and the family down in not being informed about the disability of the baby before birth. He said, "You killed me, you killed my family, we are dead."
>
> At that point I was clearly part of "the system" undifferentiated from the hospital staff whom he felt let down by. I reflected and acknowledged his anger and said: "You seem to be very angry, feel let down by everyone and might wonder if I will let you down too?" The latter part of my comment addressed the man's lack of trust towards me in the transference in a direct way, which may have helped him feel that at least I was not going to avoid painful and difficult feelings. The sense of the unknown was very powerful and included my own feelings of facing the unknown with this family, and I used this to say something about how hard and powerful it is to be suddenly faced with such an unknown painful experience as suddenly having a disabled child.

When she meets the hospital maternity team, the worker is confronted by a fresh challenge.

> The number of hospital staff involved in my various meetings with them was always surprisingly high. The hospital child protection nurse who chaired the meeting outlined their concerns, and there was particular emphasis on father's verbal violence to hospital staff and his lack of bonding with baby. From the outset all the hospital staff spoke with one voice. They were also concerned about mother not visiting during daytime or staying at night. The idea of the baby being taken into care was put forward as the solution from the very beginning.
>
> On reflection, it was as though hospital staff had made up their minds about what should happen, and my role would have been to implement their decision. By contrast, I fed back to the meeting my views about the home visit, agreed that father was clearly very angry, but thought that such a big decision might be premature for a family who are still at the early stages of coming to terms with a very traumatic event. I said "We have to give this baby and her family a chance", and that placing the baby even temporarily in care would harm the bonding relationship rather than help it.
>
> That challenge to the overriding opinion of the meeting seemed to permit some other professionals to break away from the fixed idea that placing the baby in care was the best option, and I received some support for my suggested course of action. We ended the professionals meeting deciding that there needed to be further assessment and observation of the parents' interaction with the baby and agreed to meet the next day.

From this point on, the case begins to take its more hopeful course. The worker meets daily with the family over a period of two or three weeks, father and mother start to bond well with the baby, and everyone's anxieties about risk recede. The worker is able to engage both parents in the necessary grief work associated with their loss—loss of a much-hoped-for healthy second child.

Reflecting on the process

What more can we learn from this story? Many of the same thoughts we considered in relation to the first case study apply. In effect, through astute and composed understanding of the transference forces active in the case before it has really crossed the boundary of her agency, the worker keeps her head, steadies the thinking of a complex professional system that has somewhat "lost its head" with anxiety, and establishes a therapeutic contract with a family in great distress who are at risk because a reactive professional system has stopped "thinking". When she meets the father of the family, she finds a form of words that speaks to his anger, his sense of being let down, and crucially locates herself within this transference-based interpretation—"You seem to be very angry, feel let down by everyone and might wonder if I will let you down too?"

Because she succeeds so well in staying calm and thoughtful, it becomes easy to feel critical of the hospital team, and perhaps label them risk-averse, or over-anxious. Once the social worker has got hold of her side of matters, a more balanced view would consider that different parts of the whole professional system around the family are "carrying" different aspects of the case dynamics. While the hospital team is acutely identified with the vulnerability and needs of the baby, the worker is in touch with the same qualities in the parents. The worker is more hopeful about change and the parents' potential, and the hospital more pessimistic. The case dynamics become split very quickly, and they might have remained so had the social worker not handled theses dynamics as carefully as she did. The task is to try to meet in the middle, not in a spirit of compromise, but because to make a sound assessment and decision the whole system needs to be in touch with as many dimensions of the emotional dynamics as possible.

This reflection points up how, because we are always working as a part of systems and networks, we must be capable of standing outside ourselves and seeing how we may be caught in a systemic split. Sometimes this is called occupying a "third positon". This is not easy, because the power of the feelings of identification with one or another side of a split picture can be immense. These often reflect, but are also not reducible to, a dynamic between parents or carers in the family situation. Workers make a contribution to the strong patterns of feeling and conflict that are mobilized. Roger Bacon's (1988) paper "Countertransference in a Case Conference" explores such dynamics in some depth, and Woodhouse and Pengelly's (1992) book *Anxiety and the Dynamics of Collaboration* examines how these projective and splitting processes can play out among different professions in a fixed manner, making collaboration almost impossible. Something of this is visible in the case study—the hospital team hold a conviction about the risk to the baby, but want the social worker to take on the painful and difficult task of "taking the baby into care", thus relieving them of having to think further about the case. However, the worker succeeds in handing this projection back and insisting quietly that they must all continue to think together, rather than rush to premature action.

There are real risks in becoming caught in dynamics like these. Feeling ourselves to be "recruited" or pressurized into joining the "groupthink", we will be inclined to either comply or rebel, but neither response is helpful, and it risks us losing sight of vital elements of the family's situation. The skilled use of self is, in the end, about sustaining a position of independent but connected thoughtfulness.

Conclusion—and endings

The use of self in social work is central to successful practice. Over the course of a sustained piece of work, the complexity and subtlety of the processes involved will take many forms. In more conventional therapeutic work, where there is the opportunity to maintain a stable and consistent treatment frame over a long period of time, transference and countertransference dynamics can be observed and worked with more easily than in circumstances where statutory responsibilities and anxieties are mingled with the therapeutic process. Nevertheless, when a genuine therapeutic attachment forms, it is vital not to lose sight of how significant you, the worker, become for the service user, and thus how important the ending of a piece of work will be for them.

A social worker who undertook a lengthy assessment of Anna, a young woman who had applied for a Special Guardianship order with respect to her niece, was able to explore the applicant's strengths and difficulties in depth. This was a process the young woman undoubtedly found very valuable. For example, the worker wrote:

> When Anna was able to "think" and "reflect" on her feelings and actions, she became less guarded, she opened herself to new realities, new possibilities.
>
> During session six, Anna told me that she had renewed contact with her brother whom she had not spoken to for the past two years.
>
> "I kind of realised that the reason he had not contacted me, was maybe because I had been a bit stand-offish with him, maybe he thought that I did not care, that I did not want to talk to him. Anyhow he told me he loved me at the end of his Facebook message, do you want to see it?"[2]

At the end of the assessment, the worker decides she cannot recommend Anna to be a special guardian, and clearly this affects how the process of ending the work unfolds.

> In our last two sessions, Anna appeared more guarded and less trusting, I associated this with Anna reading in my assessment my identification of her vulnerability and difficulties and her disappointment with my decision. Even though Anna was more guarded, she was able to make good use of our meetings. Mostly we explored Anna's feelings and difficulties in coming to terms with the fact that her niece was in foster care and would be adopted if Anna's appeal were not successful.
>
> I had offered to meet with Anna until the end of the court proceedings. She came to two further sessions but did not attend the subsequent ones. Somehow this felt like a natural ending. Anna was now focusing on her appeal; understandably she may have felt that communication with me may have further diminished her chances of success.

At the end of any meaningful therapeutic process, the patient or service user will often start to miss or be late for appointments. Unconsciously, perhaps, the message is, "If you can leave me, then I can do the same to you". The worker needs to stay close to her countertransference and understand that her own feelings of disappointment or frustration at missed sessions are most likely another instance of "communication by impact" or projection. A "good" ending is not necessarily a smooth or comfortable one. But as therapeutically aware social workers, we are not in the business of seeking out gratitude or emotional reward of any kind, although, of course, it is pleasing if this is conveyed. Our task is to use ourselves reflectively, maturely, and professionally.

Notes

1. The case notes in this section are from a clinical social work paper written by Ekim Erdogan in 2016 for the Tavistock Centre/UEL MA in Advanced Social Work.
2. The case notes in this section are from a clinical social work assignment written by Laura Harris in 2014 for the Tavistock Centre/UEL MA in Advanced Social Work.

CHAPTER TWO

The weight of the world: emotional and relational capacities for doing child protection work

This chapter discusses how emotions affect relationships in modern child protection work. It takes account of the nature of the task, the varying emotional capacities of practitioners, the organizational context in which the work is undertaken and managed, and the wider social and policy context, which may influence organizations and individuals.

The chapter's main themes are congruent with the comprehensive and systematically researched model of child protection work developed by Barlow and Scott (2010), in which "relational theory" informs and is informed by "relationship based practice", as central elements of the conceptual underpinning for a "21st century model of safeguarding" (p. 36). Here I focus on the experiential and relational demands of the child protection role and the associated needs of practitioners, while offering signposts to other literature that readers may wish to read in the original.

In child protection work, rapid assessments and decisions need to be made, each implying possible longer term decisions of profound and irrevocable consequence—the temporary or permanent removal of children from their families. Sometimes there are intense conflicts surrounding these actions and decisions and a reality of painful uncertainty about such decisions. Were they "right" for the child and his or her long-term future, or were the parents ultimately "right" in their desire to continue to care for their children?

In some respects "child protection" is a misleading name for the work, which always entails engagements with families, or systems of "care", within which there are vulnerable or at-risk children and young people living. Many public inquiry reports, and more recently the Munro reviews of child protection (Munro, 2010, 2011a, 2011b), have highlighted the importance of social workers' skills and confidence in relating directly to children, especially young children. But between the social worker and the child sit the adult parents and carers. Meta-analyses of Serious Case Reviews (Brandon et al., 2012) consistently reveal a trilogy of factors most frequently associated with cases of serious maltreatment—domestic violence, serious mental health problems, and drug and alcohol dependency. But whether all, or some, or none of these are features of a particular case, another factor will almost invariably be present, namely a complex, difficult, and emotionally charged set of parental or carer family histories.

And yet, people choose to do this work, sustain their commitment to it over many years, and, given the right blend of training, reflective supervision, opportunities for personal and professional development, and robust enough organizational conditions, find immense satisfaction in it—fulfilment for their sense of vocation and professional integrity. A senior practitioner in one of the teams researched by Lees (2014) commented, "You're very often taking the weight of the world on your shoulders". He was probably unaware that he was echoing the title of a book of the same name by the French sociologist Pierre Bourdieu, in which he interviewed ordinary working-class people and professionals in order to disclose the depth and intensity of "social suffering" that they bear on behalf of the rest of society, but usually without public or social recognition. Bourdieu (1999) remarked of social workers that as "agents of the state" they are "shot through with the contradictions of the state". In particular, he noted the contradiction between "the endless missions entrusted to them" and "the invariably paltry means granted to them" (p. 184).

The two primary tasks of child protection work

Child protection work is mostly undertaken beneath the surface of public or even political awareness, except, of course, on those occasions when an alleged "failure" explodes into the public and media domain. The idea that there are two "primary tasks" in child protection work, one that is about actually protecting children from harm, and another that is about protecting the rest of society from everyday awareness of the prevalence and proximity of child maltreatment, is important because it helps make sense of the continual backdrop of anxiety attending the first primary task—protecting children—which is always enacted in the shadow of the second—the fear of public humiliation, exposure, and scapegoating when a "scandal" breaks the surface. These ideas are more fully explored in Cooper (2014) but are well summarized in this quotation from an English local authority manager:

> . . . we're paid to stop the public from knowing that this sort of stuff goes on. So when the public find out about it, they get angry because they're denying that people do this stuff to children. And therefore if it becomes exposed they've got to blame somebody—"how dare you invade my living-room at six o'clock when the news is on with this horrible stuff". [Cooper & Whittaker, 2014, p. 260]

So, what makes it possible to tolerate the demands of child protection work, and even to flourish and find fulfilment in the work? The remainder of this chapter addresses this question, by keeping the experience and professional capacities of the practitioner firmly in view, but also by recognizing that contexts of practice shape experiences for better or worse.

Core skills and capacities

I propose there are a number of core relational and emotional skills and capacities required of child protection practitioners. Here, these are explored from an experiential perspective, with references to useful research and literature.

Facing difficult truths and feelings

The practitioner must have an emotional and intellectual readiness to face extremely discomforting, disturbing, emotional truths about what might be happening to children in families or other care systems, and not to turn away from feelings, signs, and observations that point towards the possibility of serious abuse. Few of us are really comfortable with the thought or the feeling that we may be in the presence of violent, damaging, sexually aggressive, or neglectful behaviour. The younger and more vulnerable the child, the more this discomfort may intensify. Equally, in relation to older children and adolescents, we may rationalize our suspicions of maltreatment by thinking of the young person as "almost an adult". This theme of both "seeing and not seeing" what is in front of our own eyes is explored in more depth in Cooper (2005b) and in M. E. Rustin (2005), two papers written in the aftermath of the Victoria Climbié inquiry in an effort to make sense of some lessons for practice and policy not addressed by the inquiry report. Cooper (2005a) and Munro (2011a) have emphasized that the question to ask is "How and why did competent people seem to have been unable to see and do the obvious in this situation?" This is a question that demands serious analytical thought, rather than a flight into blame and accusation. The answer is not straightforward and Munro's (2011a, 2011b) and others' (Stevens & Cox, 2008) discussions of "complexity" in child protection work are important. However, Burton's (2009) review of decision making and the role of supervision notes that "Managers should continuously promote an ethos of openness, rigour and challenge" in order to engage a "fresh pair of eyes" (p. 14).

Making sense of difficult experiences

The worker must have the capacity to make sense of frightening, distressing, perturbing feelings and thoughts aroused by direct contact with children and their families. Making meaning out of emotional experiences of this kind, as a way of building a picture of "what it is like for children to be inside this family" is always a provisional matter, and while it cannot usually be the only basis for decision making, it is an essential part of the process. The experience of undertaking an infant or young child observation, supported by small reflective seminar groups, is invaluable in developing this capacity for unflinching observation of both children's experience and development in a family, but also of the mind and "self" of the practitioner as she or he is emotionally engaged in intense observational and practice experiences. This method of training, originated at the Tavistock Centre in London, has formed part of some social work training in recent years, and its contribution to practitioner confidence and skills has been researched and evaluated. Urwin and Sternberg's (2012) collection offers a way into this area, with many accessible papers that describe the value of observational experience. One study of the impact of infant observation on social worker's development reported here found that at two-year follow-up, participants felt their practice had changed and that infant observation "had increased their understanding of children, families, and themselves" (p. 42).

Understanding family and system dynamics

An understanding is essential of the distinctive relational dynamics of different family systems, how these impact emotionally on the practitioner, and how inevitably she or he will be drawn into these dynamics. Systems of "care" can be thought of as lying somewhere on a spectrum. At one end are closed systems that reject help and may operate like a "gang", responding to the worker as a threatening and dangerous presence. At the other end, there may be real willingness to engage, but a sense of "stuckness" develops and the worker becomes immersed in a long relationship that feels burdensome or futile, with a powerful dynamic of aimless dependency. In between are many other possibilities, including those where parents angrily demand "help", but only on their terms, rejecting what the worker offers, until the next crisis when the pattern is repeated. Marion Bower's (2005a) paper offers a deeper account of this theme with powerful case illustrations, while Mattinson and colleagues' (1979) study of front-line practice is a neglected classic that sympathetically and vividly evokes the dynamic strains of working with difficult families. As Bower says, commenting on one case example, it is important to be aware "of the way in which the interactions of family members function as a defensive organisation, and the pressure on the social worker to enact a role which fits in with the organisation, in this case a figure who is rejecting or abusive" (Bower, 2005b, p. 159).

Building and sustaining relationships

The ability to work with and understand relationships between children and their carers, and to sustain these relationships, is obviously key. Many children who are vulnerable or at risk are not removed from their families. "Thresholds" for intervention shift constantly, and many families move back and forth between different organizational categories of concern and action. In the interests of children, the worker needs to be capable of sustaining relationships with the whole system of care, which is likely to include extended-family members and also other professionals. Tensions and conflicts about child protection interventions may be present between parents and professionals or between professionals, and resentment about continuing agency involvement is common. But such tensions are an inherent part of the "the case", and they first need to be assimilated as part of the task if they are to be constructively tackled. A central source of tension in worker–family relationships is the fact that many carers of children at risk are perfectly aware of the inadequacy of their parenting, but feel profoundly guilty or ashamed, intensely vulnerable to criticism, and they fear the consequences of professional involvement. They may not find it easy to admit their anxieties to themselves, let alone to a child protection practitioner who may exercise statutory authority and holds power over family life.

To be curious about the family story

A simple way of starting to manage parents' and carers' anxieties about their own care and about the reality of professional involvement, as well as gaining vital understanding of the meaning of any suspected abuse, is for the worker to be curious and enquiring about the parents' or carers' own stories of their childhoods and parenting. All parents have a story. To show genuine curiosity about these histories, is not to evade the need for a focus on the welfare of the children, except in circumstances of emergency. Rather, it is to engage the carers in a process of empathic "sense making" of the very situation that has brought them to professional attention. Once revealed, the links between how abusive or neglectful parents relate to their children, and how they were parented themselves, are frequently striking and transparent to everyone. But often no one has previously thought to ask and to encourage reflection on these. The power of the "ghosts" that haunt the family script and the transformative potential of exploring these is wonderfully articulated in Fraiberg, Adelson, and Shapiro's classic (1975) paper. A focus on children as a part of their families, rather than just the child, is part of the "relational" model advocated by Barlow and Scott (2010).

Using reflective supervision: the importance of containment

In my experience, any group of social workers discussing their work and organizations will soon enough turn to the question of supervision. A lack of reflective supervision focused on understanding the case and the emotional and relational challenges it presents, the encroachment of "managerial" supervision on the reflective space, and the decline in supervisory skills among social work managers are some of the most pressing issues for contemporary child protection practice. Part One of the *Munro Review of Child Protection* is strong on this point and notes that, "To work with families with compassion but retain an open and questioning mindset requires regular, challenging supervision. The emotional and intellectual demands on social workers are substantial; this and their need for high quality supervision and support has been accepted by the Social Work Task Force" (Munro, 2010, p. 18).

Toasland's (2007) paper addresses the important link between the positive emotional and relational conditions that support children's healthy development and the parallel provision of reflective and containing supervision for professionals working with parents who may not be able to offer this, and who may not have received it themselves. "Containment" is the interpersonal, psychological process of receiving difficult, anxious, disturbing, or unacceptable emotional communications from another person, tolerating them, becoming able to think about them, and then finding ways to resume communication with the other person so that, for them, these states of mind become, in turn, more manageable, tolerable, and "thinkable". Many of the children with whom child protection practitioners work have not enjoyed a reliable or consistent-enough experience of this kind with their parents or carers, who in turn have often been denied it for themselves, and thus transfer their struggle on to professionals, and not necessarily with awareness. Such unprocessed emotional communication is contagious, in the sense that it may be transmitted from person to person until someone succeeds in making emotional and cognitive sense of the feelings and thoughts involved—or not. While Toasland's (2007) paper on the importance of social work management providing "containment for the container" is a helpful point of entry to this area, because front-line child protection work, via processes of projection of the kind just outlined, often leaves practitioners feeling ashamed, as though it is *they* who are inadequate, blameworthy, failing, wrong, and even abusive, seeking supervisory help is not always straightforward. None of us are likely to be comfortable at revealing such anxieties, self-doubt, and erosion of self-confidence to a colleague, especially a manager. In my experience of training with experienced practitioners, it is the provision of non-judgemental, thoughtful, small-group "work-discussion" spaces (Rustin & Bradley, 2008) that they find most valuable in "detoxifying" their experience of the work. Agency provision of good supervision is vital, but reluctance to avail oneself of it may be as important in its breakdown as managerial neglect, and so the "management" of supervision must take account of this dynamic.

Managing in relation to your colleagues and agency

From my experience, an unacknowledged truth about most people's working lives is that what keeps them awake at night is tensions and conflicts with colleagues and managers, as much as anxiety about the work itself. Child protection workers do carry a continual burden of worry about their caseloads, and their organizational worries add to this. There is a long and helpful tradition of research and writing that tries to understand the nature of organizational tensions and conflicts by looking at how these mirror or represent "enactments" of the conflicts and anxieties present in the dynamics of the service-user systems themselves (e.g., Bacon, 1988; Mattinson et al., 1979), as well as how systematic defences arise in organizations to protect staff from too much anxiety about the work. Recent studies of child protection teams (Lees, 2014; Whittaker, 2011) show that "delegation upwards" from front-line staff to managers is a common defence, allowing workers to sidestep the anxiety of decision making while radically eroding their sense of autonomy, discretion, and scope for professional judgement. Andrew Whittaker's 2011 paper, in which he discusses a "practice-near" ethnographic study of four front-line child protection teams, is a very helpful introduction to this way of thinking, but, as discussed above, see also Lees (2014) and Cooper and Lees (2014) for accounts that offer insight into the challenges that modern organizational cultures pose for child protection practitioners in realizing their potential as autonomous professionals.

At the "front line"

I shall pause here to think about the language we deploy in discussing child protection work. The "front line", "bombardment", "siege mentality", and many other common metaphors speak to an underlying sense of this work as akin to war, as Beckett (2003) has noted. But we should surely be reflective and questioning about our discourses, otherwise they inhabit us, and we them, in an uncritical way and this constrains our capacity for "agency", our ability to take more charge of the work and our experience of it, rather than it controlling us. Child protection work may feel like a war zone sometimes, but it is not war. To forget this is to forget that its aim is ultimately benign and reparative: to protect children and help struggling parents and carers with the most important "task" any of us assume in our lives.

I wish to comment on a passage drawn from a research interview that is part of a doctoral project for which I am the supervisor that aims to record the emotional realities of front-line workers' experiences and states of mind (Noyes, 2015). By way of background, the very experienced social worker, who is the respondent in the research interview, describes in her own words what is it like to work with a young mother of a 2-year-old child on a child protection plan for eighteen months or so. The worker's name has been changed to Kate for purposes of confidentiality. I suggest that this research interview excerpt shows the vividness of language that the practitioner searches for in order to convey to the research interviewer how she has experienced elements of her contact with the mother. I would also like to draw attention to the importance of a receptive, listening *supervisory-type* presence to allow the worker to communicate her experience.

Case excerpt

INTERVIEWER: And you're doing a kind of sucking motion with your mouth . . .

SOCIAL WORKER: Yes well . . . she sort of sucks the life out of you and I (*laughs*) have to go, and just getting her to sort of . . . it has been a struggle. I've worked with her now . . . for eighteen months, just over eighteen months and . . . there have been visits when I have been talking about really serious concerns around relationships with her partner and issues around the child protection plan . . . and I just think "Am I getting through to you?" How am I communicating with you? But I go away thinking . . . I get in the car and I go . . . oh . . .

INTERVIEWER: And you're bodily showing me that you sag.

SOCIAL WORKER: Yes, (*raises voice*) I do sag and I just think oh goodness me, and I sort of go ooh . . . do that with my head sort of shaking my head and I just think did I get through to her at all and as I say, it can be really difficult things or it can be really positive things I'm going with, and I still can get the same response.

It did very much feel like I was talking to myself over and over and saying the same thing. That's quite disheartening going every visit, sometimes two, three times a week when it's really serious and saying the same thing over and over again but (*hits table/chair*) reflecting back I think "Well, actually all that hard work you put in with her, Kate, has paid off because some of it must have soaked

> in because she's changed slowly by slowly maybe at her own pace but she has actually made progress really" but . . . and I like her, I do like her, I've got a lot of empathy and sympathy for her. You know, I feel quite sorry for her because . . . with her experiences and her child . . . and I think she wants to be nurtured by me as well and sort of give her the positives and nurture and that's been a resistance in me because I'm *not* her mum and um don't want to be put into the mum role—it's a sort of carrot and stick with her all the time.

What can we notice about this social worker's narration of her experience in the context of a research interview? There is a whole dimension of the worker's communications to the researcher that are not just non-verbal, but are actively expressed through bodily gestures—sighs, sagging, sucking, hitting the table. The researcher can be seen, in the interview transcript, reflecting back to the worker her impressions of the worker's body language as she, the worker, recounts experiences of working with this young mother. What I see in this research interview is an example of the components of receptive, listening *supervisory-type* presence.

My further observation of this account within the research transcript is that whole areas of the young woman's emotional experience cannot be communicated in a way that the worker can fully understand or fully make sense of. The language used and her actions suggest to me a worker who is stuck, a case that is emotionally stuck, despite the fact that there is engagement between the mother and the worker and some progress described in the case. The sense of "banging one's head against a brick wall" is not just spoken about but conveyed in the narration itself: the emphatic repetition of *serious*, the *same*, *every*, *nothing*, and so on possibly impacts on the listener to produce the same effect the young woman has had on the worker—a kind of deadening of the relationship, maybe.

The worker is aware of being drawn into a "mothering" role despite herself, such is the power of the essentially unconscious communications to which she is subject. It seems the young mother cannot really talk *about* certain aspects of her own experience, especially of her childhood and parenting, but I would suggest they are re-enacted with the worker. These unconscious communications take root in the worker as bodily experiences that are weighing her, the worker, down. I think the research interviewer does a simple but skilled job of mirroring these unconscious processes back to the worker.

Responsibility, anxiety, and defences

Skilled and experienced child protection practitioners carry an immense weight of responsibility for their work and live with anxiety about the decisions they must make that concern the temporary or permanent removal of a child, about the risks to children on their caseloads who may remain inadequately protected over time, and about the suffering that children are enduring. Often practitioners are frightened, because a proportion of families with whom they work have members who are threatening, violent, and dangerous, and these cases exert a disproportionate influence on the mind and work of child protection practitioners. These professionals need and deserve confident and sustained organizational support in order to sustain their ability to do the work over long time periods, to maintain professional confidence in themselves, and for the well-being of the children and families with whom they work. Their organizations and managers are frequently under economic pressure, and a range of expectations bear down on modern public services which often seem to be making good practice harder, while claiming to do the opposite—harsh and arbitrary performance and inspection regimes, unrealistic time scales for assessment and decision making, efficiency, and productivity targets, which are often euphemisms for resource reductions, as well as perpetual "churn" in the policy environment.

These external factors, which occasion organizational anxiety and defensiveness because they can be experienced as a threat to organizational survival or credibility, often intersect with the anxieties arising from the primary task itself to produce a particular fear-laden "structure of feeling" in child protection services that is indeed challenging. Cooper and Lees (2014), drawing on the tradition of thinking originated by Menzies Lyth about social systems as a defence against anxiety (Menzies, 1959), as well as recent research into the emotional life of front-line child protection teams, argue that modern organizational contexts generate new forms of professional anxiety. The nurses and nurse managers in Menzies Lyth's original study of a general hospital were shown to be anxious about the potential for physical and emotional harm to patients entailed by their routine tasks. Defensive behaviours against this anxiety often took the form of "ritual task performance" and "upward delegation" of decision making and responsibility, in a way that became formally inscribed in the organizational system. Lees' (2014) research revealed similar patterns of anxiety and defensiveness in child protection teams, but in addition the impact of inspection regimes and performance management targets also gave rise to intense anxiety, not about "doing harm" to service users, but about external judgements of professional failure, incompetence, or culpability that might result in injury to the professional "self" of the workers and their organizations. These two forms of anxiety are different in important ways, but the defensive behaviours elaborated to cope with them had very similar qualities. Cooper and Lees (2014; see also chapter 4 herein) comment:

> Hence the familiar and oft-repeated observations about contemporary defensive organizational practices being directed towards "covering your back". What is implicitly lamented here is precisely the replacement of concern (albeit anxious concern) for the patient or service user, by a dominant anxiety for the survival of the professional self. [Cooper & Lees, 2014, p. 244]

Final observation

In an important paper, mentioned earlier, the American social worker and therapist Selma Fraiberg evoked the idea of "ghosts in the nursery", the emotionally active residues of parents' own difficult childhood experiences that are revisited on their children in turn (Fraiberg, Adelson, & Shapiro, 1975). Ghosts in the nursery are a universal experience, as Fraiberg makes plain, but in certain cases cannot be laid to rest. In such cases, the child protection worker becomes the latest recipient of a visitation from these "ghosts", who take up residence in the workers' bodies and minds in disturbing, perplexing, and burdensome ways. But this can only happen if the worker is first of all available to create a relationship in which this can happen. This is step one. Step two is about making sense of these communications with the help of others, and, finally, step three is the skill of making use of new understanding about family relationships to start a process of change in these relationships. Sometimes this is not possible even with specialized therapeutic input, and then begins the difficult task of assessing whether the right course of action in the child's long-term interests may be removal.

This brings us more or less full circle, to some of the core dilemmas of child protection work outlined at the start of the chapter. The "weight of the world" cannot always be allowed to remain with the child, and so it passes to us as members of the child protection system to assume responsibility for it, as best we can.

PART II

ORGANIZATIONS

CHAPTER THREE

Legend, myth, and idea: on the fate of a great paper

Introduction: legend and myth

Isabel Menzies Lyth's seminal paper on social systems as a defence against anxiety (Menzies, 1959) is so well known and frequently cited that it risks acquiring mythic or legendary status. But what explains its phenomenal influence? In this chapter, I suggest that it is a model example of the psychoanalytic case study, deriving its power from a deep engagement with organizational particularities as a basis for general theorizing. Its continued influence depends upon the way in which it is used to conceptualize new organizational experiences. An example from an institutional observation undertaken as part of an advanced social work training at the Tavistock illustrates this. Institutional observation is one of a range of non-clinical psychoanalytically informed methods of training at the Tavistock, and in the final part of the chapter I discuss new applications of Menzies Lyth's work that aim to illuminate the irrational forces shaping modern social policy.

Modern organizational anxieties are discussed in much greater detail in the next chapter of this book, and the original paper on which the present chapter is based was my first attempt to formulate these. Death, and anxieties about death, emerge as a subtext of this discussion, perhaps reflecting the fact that the original paper was prepared as part of a memorial conference to Menzies Lyth herself, and also that her paper taught us to think better about death as an aspect of organizational experience.

How many of us can name more than one paper written by Isabel Menzies Lyth, and how many can provide the title of that one paper fully and accurately? *That* paper. It's a bit like *The Communist Manifesto*. Within our admittedly rather small and esoteric community, it is *so* famous that it is in danger of acquiring modern celebrity status—that is, of being famous for being famous—while being properly read by a declining group of people. What a terrible fate.

Organizational case studies

Why has it acquired such status? Psychoanalysis is built upon a foundation of individual case studies—Freud's Wolf Man or his Little Hans, Klein's Richard, and so on. I believe that when the single case study works, it does so because it captures the deep particularity of that case and, simultaneously, shows us how it necessarily partakes of the universal, general, or invariant principles of which the case is a unique instance. In this way, the good case study embodies a paradox. Great case studies work in the same way as great novels or poems. If a case study achieves this kind of stature, then time, social change, new theoretical developments, and so forth do not invalidate its core of validity, despite the fact that it will come to seem dated. "A Case Study in the Functioning of Social Systems as a Defence against Anxiety" (Menzies, 1959) does seem dated now, and I believe this is partly because the nature of organizations in our society has changed sufficiently since its publication for us to need to stand back and ask, "Do we need to revise the theoretical precepts that inform this great paper, and which it also generated" (Cooper & Dartington, 2004).

As I thought about the various ways in which I wanted to explore this question to which the answer is both "yes" and "no", I found that most of what I wanted to say was about death. Perhaps that is apposite in a whole number of ways, just one of which is that, as mentioned above, the paper was prepared for a memorial conference to commemorate the life and work of Isabel Menzies Lyth. Perhaps people, or at least some people, die differently now from how they did in 1960. But as Ludwig Wittgenstein (1974, p. 72,) once observed, "Death is not an event in life: we do not live to experience death."

Death and the organization

So, first, the particularity of the case study method. Students who undertake institutional observations within the Tavistock tradition do so in the benign shadow of Menzies Lyth's paper—and will always do so, I suspect. Task-related anxiety, and defences against it, is one key idea you want the student to get hold of through observation, and to get hold of through *experience*. If a student does not have the opportunity to undertake a personal analysis or therapy as part of a course or training, the Tavistock tradition has devised all sorts of pretty good substitutes—group relations events, infant observation, experiential groups, and institutional observations. A post-qualifying social work student decided to undertake his institutional observation by attending Sunday morning meetings at his local Quaker meeting house. He describes how often, in the silence of the meeting, his thoughts turned to death. He wonders why this should be, and then at one point, reflecting partly on the age of the majority of those attending, he asks himself whether this non-proselytizing religious institution might harbour unconscious anxieties about its own capacity to survive.

> During my observations individuals felt moved to share poems or lines from the bible:
>
> > *He read aloud the poem "This Was The Summer Day" by Mary Oliver which ended with the line "Tell me, what is it you plan to do with your one wild and precious life . . ." I felt suddenly wonderfully positive and wanted to clap. No one said anything or moved and he sat back down and closed his eyes. I thought "Yes, what am I to do with my one precious life?" Any thoughts of death or dying suddenly left me. (Week 4)*
>
> This felt to me to be an attempt to challenge the "deadliness" which existed in the group, an attempt to bring life back into the organization. The Quakers have a long and proud tradition of pacifism and non-intervention, they are against wars, but does this become a form of death in itself? I felt myself anxious on behalf of these gentle people who seemed unable to "save their own lives", I became worried about whether they could save their organization? Hopes for the future focused in my mind on a young boy who attended the group with his mother:
>
> > *The four-year-old boy I had noticed before sat next to his mother. He looked around the group fidgeted on his seat and whispered to his mother. He then silently started counting by pointing at everyone as he*

> *went round the circle. I smiled because this is often what I did during observations—without pointing. (Week 9)*
>
> *The four-year-old stood up and took his mother's hand. They both left to go to another room next door. I felt sad as they left as all life seemed to leave the room. (Week 9)*

> It seemed significant in my mind that the young boy could not stand the "deadly" silence for long periods and left after only ten or fifteen minutes of the group meeting to play next door. As the youngest member, it also felt to me as if life was leaving the room as he left.
>
> The endings of the meetings were almost as enigmatic to me as the start or the content. As I entered the room the group were already in silence, nobody ever said "*right we are all silent now, so say nothing*". For all I knew as I entered it felt as if they could have been sitting in the meeting room all night. It was almost as if the sudden ending was like a death itself, a sudden inexplicable change in the group:
>
> > *Suddenly a woman in her early 60s, who looked like an ex-headteacher stood up and everyone moved. I was taken aback at the sudden movement, which seemed out of keeping from the previous hour's silence. (Week 1)*[1]

Psychoanalytic therapy is largely, in my view, the practice of helping people think thoughts that have hitherto been too painful or difficult to bear. To do this the therapist must first be able to bear the unbearable thoughts and feelings in that field of experience we call the countertransference. We often refer to this function or practice as "containment". I think Isabel Menzies Lyth taught us that institutions are asked to perform a similar kind of work on behalf of their members, and for society more generally, and that like therapists—or anyone, in fact—they sometimes do it well and sometimes not so well, and sometimes they need help with the difficulty of the task. The thought that you may be dying as an institution after some hundreds of years may just not be thinkable.

This student did not know until I told him that there is more than a coincidental connection between the practices of Quaker meetings and the teaching and learning methods of the Tavistock Centre. In his paper on this theme, "The Quaker Connection in the Tavistock Clinic's development", Sebastian Kraemer says:

> When I arrived at the Tavistock Clinic as a psychiatric registrar over thirty years ago I remember thinking that the reflective practice of

> seminars, including the arrangement of chairs in a circle, might be something like a Quaker meeting, though I had never (and still have not) been to one. Only recently did it occur to me that there may actually be a connection. It turned out there was more than I expected. [2011, p. 82]

He later quotes from a lecture by John Rickman, one of the analysts who influenced those who shaped Tavistock methods, about the Quakers:

> There is an element of mutual admiration and a tendency to undue exaltation of the performances of the members or of the group as a whole, but there is another and more valuable process at work as well: the production of an atmosphere of tolerance towards the expression of any idea irrespective of the effect that the idea may have on the individual or on society. I do not want to minimise the dangers of this atmosphere . . . [Rickman, 2003, p. 287]

The "dangers of this atmosphere" when applied to the study of institutions are equally not to be minimized, and I have known observers (not just 4-year-old children) to find it impossible for one reason or another to see through the task of simply sitting and bearing their emotional experience in an organization for one hour. But whatever is learned about an organization's anxieties and methods of defending itself against anxiety via this method, I want to stress that what it gives access to is the very *particular* nature of the *particular* organization under study. We cannot jump to the conclusion that, for example, it is a function of all organized religious institutions to contain or manage anxieties about dying on behalf of the wider society, although, as I shall explore a little later, this may not be a completely silly hypothesis.

Modern anxieties

I have said that maybe the model of organizations implied by Menzies Lyth's paper might stand in need of revision. I briefly want to explore why, although the argument is elaborated more fully in chapter 4. I am indebted to my colleague Tony McCaffrey for the following succinct and original way of telling the changing story of anxiety in human service organizations over the last twenty or thirty years.

The story begins with the familiar idea for which we are indebted to Menzies Lyth—the organization as container of professional anxiety arising from the nature of the primary task. Strong systems for the provision of reflective supervision to front-line staff might be part of this picture. But at a certain juncture, in the 1980s perhaps, new forms of anxiety begin to bear down on institutions. "Rationing anxiety" arises as our leaders and politicians lose faith in the limitless capacity of the state to fund health and social welfare in this country—people are living longer, the proportionate tax base to fund pensions and the economically inactive is shrinking, medical technologies are proving expensive as well as effective, leading to a growing population of ageing citizens—and in recognition of these developments, or perhaps emphasizing them at the expense of seeking state-funded solutions to them, new ideologies of welfare and health provision make their appearance. The tension that begins to appear is well illustrated in a story told by Tony McCaffrey (personal communication). He was consulting to a group of managers in a north London hospital, struggling with the impact of cost savings, so that acute-bed spaces are full to overflowing. There was a serious road accident on a nearby busy highway, and a patient was flown into the hospital by air ambulance. The A&E manager arrives late to the consultancy group as a result, relates this story, and adds, "But fortunately, the patient was dead on arrival".

Then markets or quasi-markets make their appearance in the public sector, and in their wake comes the whole panoply of performance management systems, audit and inspection regimes, and regulatory practices, with which we are all familiar. These are designed to ensure that standards are being maintained and "value for money" extracted from our services. New forms of survival anxiety appear—less directly associated with money, more with quality and the measurement of quality. For short, I call this "performance anxiety". As the imperative towards a mixed economy of care evolves in tandem with the new commissioner–provider split, compulsory competitive tendering and "contestability", then traditional boundaries between different sectors of provision—public, private, independent—become blurred. Services are delivered via partnerships, networks, and multi-agency systems, and frequently no one seems to have single overall control or authority within these systems. The peculiarly named phenomenon of "governance" appears in an effort to provide some form of order in the face of the potential chaos of these new systems, many of which operate at arm's length from the state. "Partnership" or "governance anxiety" is added to the gallery (see Figure 3.1). In chapter 4, I describe how, in the wake of the economic crisis of 2008, organizational "survival anxiety" takes its place alongside these accumulating forms of contemporary organizational anxiety.

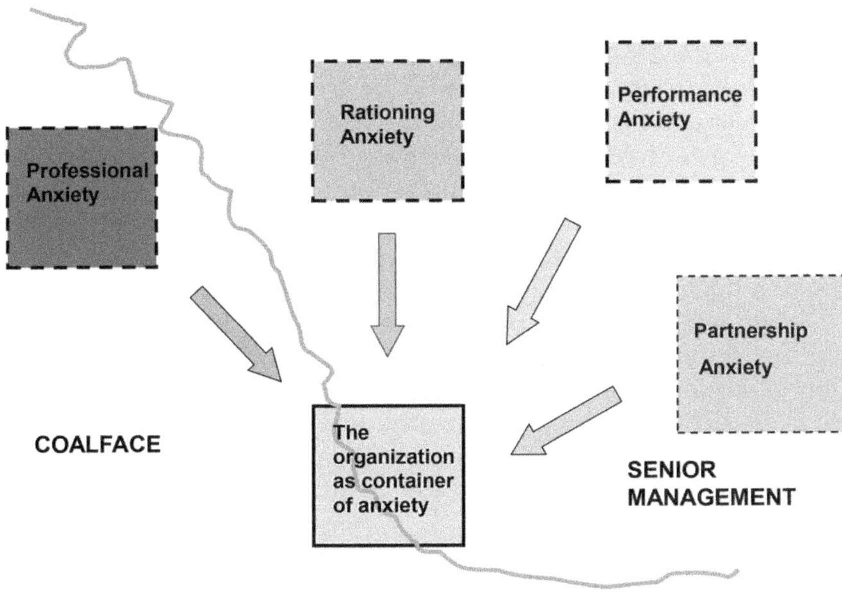

Figure 3.1. Anxiety in organizations—a history. (With acknowledgements to Tony McCaffrey.)

Increasingly, a fracture appears within organizations; senior and middle managers face "outwards" in their effort to manage the demands of cost, competition, performance, and partnership, leaving front-line staff isolated in their struggle with the face-to-face task, which in truth may not have changed that much. Most first-line and middle managers to whom I have shown the diagram in Figure 3.1 seem to recognize the picture—more than one has said something like, "I walk along that jagged line every day".

My question is: in the face of this story, does the traditional psychoanalytic story of organizational anxiety and defences against anxiety need some modification? I believe it does. Or perhaps it always did present a rather too-neat and simple account of how anxieties are generated and contained (or not) in organizations. Perhaps the emotional life of organizations always was rather more politically and socially inflected than we recognized? But once again, perhaps the great and illuminating case study works precisely *because* it does edit out complexity, or "noise", leaving us with a kind of ideal type or "pure culture" of the phenomenon being studied.

Whatever, I seem to be proposing that we cannot any more usefully model the nature of the emotional life of organizations without attention to the impact of the policy and political environment. So can Isabel Menzies Lyth help us with this re-modelling? I think she can. Another great strength of the central idea about task, anxiety, and social systems as a defence against anxiety is how widely—not to say sometimes wildly—and generally applicable it seems to be. *Anything*, one suddenly realizes, that looks remotely like a social system or social process might actually be functioning as a defence against anxiety.

Now, this has given rise to some wonderfully exciting and, I believe, important ideas, even if they are ideas that are very difficult to evidence in a systematic way, although the empirical research discussed in chapter 4 is one attempt to ground this thesis in good evidence. In his chapter "Managing Social Anxieties in Public Sector Organizations", Anton Obholzer wrote the following, now quite famous, words:

> In the unconscious, there is no such concept as "health". There is, however, a concept of "death", and in our constant attempt to keep this anxiety repressed, we use various unconscious defensive mechanisms, including the creation of social systems to serve the defensive function. Indeed our health service might more accurately be called a keep-death-at-bay-service. [Obholzer, 1994, p. 171]

If this is the case, can we in any way explain what sometimes seems to be a determined effort to ruin our health service via the imposition of efficiency savings, targets, audit, performance-management regimes, and so on? Is the collective unconscious somehow sabotaging itself? Maybe so, and I will conclude with a few thoughts on this.

But first let me give some personal observational evidence for Obholzer's thesis. It was my misfortune to be admitted to hospital with a nasty infection that had got out of control. In retrospect, I think I was pretty anxious about the whole experience. I spent a lot of time closely observing the institutional processes around me, and sometimes being inflicted upon me. Presumably, this is a case of the functioning of institutional observation as a defence against anxiety. It did seem to me that the many, many systems that go to make up the total life of the hospital ward were hopelessly ill coordinated. Nursing, catering, cleaning, pharmaceutical, infection control, and medical systems seemed to intersect terribly poorly, and within themselves, to effect very poor handovers between shifts. I observed a patient being admitted to our ward late at night and later his relative asking him the whereabouts of his hearing aid. After his relative had gone, a nurse appeared and began to ask him questions. After a while I did intervene and say, "I think this man wears a hearing aid", and she thanked me. But next morning this information seemed to have been lost as another clinician struggled to communicate with her patient. I gave up trying to solve all the systemic problems around me and settled for trying to be a patient myself, though clearly, as my fellow patient answered yes or no to questions from doctors that I thought he could not hear, this loss of information in the system was potentially dangerous to him.

Death made its appearance in the following way: another man was transferred into our little six-bed ward space late one night as I was trying to sleep. Then I heard his wife come beetling down the corridor, saying "Are you alright now? I'll see you in the morning . . ." "Is there any chance of a drop of water?" said the man. "No, no, you're in the hospital now, you can't have any water", said his wife. "Ah well," came the reply, "a man could feckin' die in here then."

With a number of colleagues, I have been teaching psychoanalytically informed social policy to our social work students at the Tavistock for the last few years. In truth, given that there is not much of a tradition of such work (but see chapters 10 and 11), we and the students have largely been making it up as we go along. Isabel Menzies Lyth has, for better or worse, been our constant companion on this voyage. Modern social work is deeply impacted by what seem, intuitively, to be anxious social and political responses to evidence of risk, failure, and damage in our society. Interrogated from this kind of perspective, many of the all too familiar instruments of modern social policy—regimes of audit, inspection, regulation, procedure, risk management, and so on—themselves turn out (on closer inspection, as it were) to have something to do with an effort to ward off death, or the fear of death, or the fear of being blamed for death. "We must ensure this is never allowed to happen again" is the common political response to the emergence into public awareness of a new tragedy. "And to ensure this never happens again, my civil servants will write some new procedures" is what usually ensues. I believe a large part of this superstructure of inspection and checking is actually a form of ritual, and that those who administer it are priests of the various churches that have grown up to help us manage our anxieties about death in a secular age.

It might be a surprising thought that the contradictions of modern social policy can be partly explained by their "excess rationality", which in turn might derive from contemporary misconceptions about the nature of (social) science, society itself, and their relationship to faith, including religious faith. But if so, then so much the better, for we need a world full of surprises. The philosopher and literary critic Terry Eagleton has given voice to some of what I am hinting at here:

> A society of packaged fulfilment, administered desire, managerialized politics, and consumerist economics is unlikely to cut to the kind of depth where theological questions can even be properly raised, just as it rules out political and moral questions of a certain profundity. [Eagleton, 2009, p. 39]

So, here is a little meta-theoretical support for a grand, if so far rather loosely elaborated thesis about modern social and political formations, and their relationship to primitive anxieties and to our unconscious fear of death, the same fear that my student detected under the surface of the religious organization he was observing. Whether you buy it or not, I think it is a pretty interesting idea. It is an idea that could not, in my view, ever have been born without the great and important ideas forged from the close study of particular organizational experience contained in the Menzies Lyth paper—that is part of her legacy to us.

Note

1. From an unpublished institutional observation paper written in 2008 by Stephen Jordan at the Tavistock Clinic and University of East London.

CHAPTER FOUR

Spotlit: defences against anxiety in contemporary human service organizations

Introduction

Why is statutory child protection such a fraught and conflicted organizational activity? This chapter aims to shed light on some key dimensions of twenty-first century organizational life that help provide an answer, and it takes child protection work as its main case study. Chapter 2 of this book engages with some of the same ideas in a more practical and immediate way, as part of a discussion about the key professional capacities required to survive and flourish as a modern child protection worker. Chapter 3 provides a backdrop to the specific thesis elaborated in this chapter about the distinctively contemporary character of lived working experience in human service organizations.

Organizational formations and cultures in the twenty-first century are in rapid and radical evolution. However, trajectories of change differ according to political, social, and cultural contexts. In British

An earlier version of this chapter was published as A. Cooper & A. Lees, "Spotlit: Defences against Anxiety in Contemporary Human Service Organizations", in D. Armstrong & M. Rustin (Eds.), *Social Defences against Anxiety: Explorations in a Paradigm* (London: Karnac, 2014).

public sector contexts the influence of neo-liberal market ideologies and practices, encapsulated by New Public Management theory, may be a dominant transnational force intersecting with other local and national traditions and trends. Isabel Menzies Lyth's original thesis about the functioning of social systems as a defence against anxiety (Menzies, 1959) was itself developed under specific professional and historical circumstances and is also imbued with particular psychoanalytic theoretical presuppositions.

In this chapter, I propose that the meaningful application of her ideas to contemporary human and public service organizations requires considerable development of the precepts shaping the founding thesis. First, in summary, the nature and sources of the anxieties with which front-line staff and human service managers must contend have evolved to include a powerful range of extra-organizational forces and pressures; second, the anxieties arising from these new sources are typically different from the familiar task-related anxieties that were Menzies Lyth's main preoccupation, but they are also often congruent with the latter in important ways. I suggest it is helpful to think of task-related anxieties as predominantly "depressive" in nature—that is, entailing anxiety about the potential to cause harm or injury to vulnerable service users and patients—and those emanating from the managerial and political environment as predominantly "persecutory"—that is, entailing threats of harm to the self of the worker. Both varieties of anxiety give rise to socially structured defences, and both also generate "secondary anxieties" which are the unintended consequences of these defences.

A nuanced capacity to disentangle these different processes, and their effects on organizational experience, is required. So third, the contemporary state of affairs requires a more fully psycho-social framework of understanding than Menzies Lyth offered, in which there is (at least) a two-way direction of influence acting on operatives to produce their "lived experience" of the work and its organizational context. The total situation results in a distinctive "structure of feeling" characterized by "fear and dread" in modern British human services. This overall way of thinking indicates a need for case-study–based research programmes that capture the particularities of specific organizational/cultural formations. The chapter reports and draws upon the findings of a small-scale ethnographic empirical study of front-line child protection services to elaborate and illustrate this wider thesis.

The transformation of human service organizations

In chapter 3, I suggested that since the 1980s British public sector organizations have been the object of successive but also cumulative waves of external pressure associated with the neo-liberal political project and its determination to variously "transform", shrink, marketize, or reposition the welfare state as a whole in its relation to wider economic and state–civil society boundaries. "Modernization" is often the catch-all phrase for these trends, although this term may disguise as much as it reveals about the deep structure of the transformations concerned. Resource rationing, performance management and target cultures, inspection and audit regimes associated with a "value-for-money" public transparency and choice ethic, interagency and cross-sector collaboration ("joined-up working"), all combine to create a distinctive and new network of organizational demands, accompanied by new forms of professional anxiety. In many ways, these contextual forces constitute the phenomenon of public sector "governance", itself a telling neologism denoting a variety of social order and discipline unsteadily located on the boundary between traditional government and new forms of regulation and social surveillance.

Hoggett (2010) and others suggest that the distorting impact of these forces in relation to the traditionally conceived "primary tasks" of health and care services constitutes a kind of systematic perversion of those tasks. Krantz (2010) points to the influence of new technologies and digital information and communication systems as further transformative forces shaping organizational life, mobilizing new and unfamiliar forms of anxiety. To date, however, there has been little empirical study of whether and how professional anxieties have actually been modified by these developments, or whether we can confidently assert the emergence of new forms of defence against such anxieties. Anecdotal and experiential accounts abound, but the danger here is that we narrate and hear only those anecdotes that confirm our fears and anxieties about social change, so that the important project of describing and conceptualizing change processes becomes confused with a "narrative of loss".

The research project described below was undertaken by Amanda Lees, and in part it set out to test the validity of Andrew Cooper's and others' formulations about modern organizational anxieties (Lees, 2014). However, the two authors did not collaborate on this project, and they only met one another after it had been written up. This work describes in detail organizational structures and systems, behaviours, practices, rituals, and affective states that will seem very familiar to anyone who has a working relationship with modern British health or statutory-care settings. Alongside a necessarily summary account of this work, the chapter offers some additional anecdotal accounts of direct experiences of the contemporary "structure of feeling" in these settings, because it is important to grasp just how extreme these can be, and thus how important it is to achieve a more coherent and convincing understanding of what is being enacted in the name of "care" or "welfare" in our society—and what part "defences against anxiety" play in all this.

Cases and contexts

The theoretical ambivalence of Menzies Lyth, Elliott Jaques, and others towards the ontological autonomy of defensive systems at the organizational or cultural levels is more fully explored in Cooper (1996). William Halton (2014) has suggested that the defences against anxiety reported by Menzies Lyth in her original study are obsessional in nature, and this resonates with my contemporary experience, with earlier theorizations set out in Cooper and Lousada (2005), and with Amanda Lees's new findings. Like Halton, I think it important to be able to specify the anxieties that might be shaping any particular organizational culture, and I have some propositions to advance about the specific nature of task-related anxieties in the care and health sector, and societal anxieties that intersect with these.

The specificities of context-shaping organizational cultures and anxieties, allied to the differential nature of organizational primary tasks which are assumed to mobilize anxieties, suggest that a rigorous case study approach is required for the development of both more refined theory and useful models to inform consultancy or other practical interventions. As Obholzer (1989) notes, Menzies Lyth's key propositions include that "there is innate psychic pain inherent in all institutions [and] that the nature of the pain is specific to the primary task of the institutions". Given the additional variable of social–political context, what holds for a financial services organization in Hong Kong will probably not hold for a hospice in Harrow. Differential organizational forms, the characteristic anxieties their tasks generate, the societal pressures and demands shaping their evolution, distinctive professional cultures within a society, and so on, all combine to create particular organizational "cases" which must be understood psycho-socially as "complex particulars" (see chapter 12). Different organizational cases may manifest considerable similarities with one another, but complex particularity means that these will take the form of stronger or weaker "family resemblances" rather than simply identity or difference.

The case of English child protection work

Amanda Lees's (2014) study was undertaken in three systemically linked front-line child protection teams in an English local authority, with a focus on information-sharing practices. We suggest that English child protection organizations, policies, and practices over the last decade provide unusually instructive examples of how task-related anxieties and internally generated organizational responses to these have intersected in complex and unpredictable ways with powerful political, cultural, and societal processes, to produce organizational "states of mind" consistent with those described by Menzies Lyth, but not actually explicable solely in terms of the mechanisms she postulates.

Rigidly protocolized information-sharing practices are a salient feature of this picture. Overtly, these new procedures and practices derive from the repeated findings of public inquiries, Serious Case Reviews, and other analyses of "failures to protect" children at risk that ineffective information sharing among agencies and between intra-agency subsystems made a significant contribution to the ultimate fate of children at risk. However, the organizational mind states and behaviours associated with these practices bear all the hallmarks of a socially constructed system of defences, with the "obsessional" features noted by William Halton very much in evidence. But what accounts for what in this picture? Do profound task-related anxieties associated with professional responsibility for "safeguarding" vulnerable and at-risk children from harm, and ultimately death, dispose front-line and first-line managerial staff to erect organizational systems of defence? Or do public, judicial, and media allegations against individuals, organizations, and at times entire professions of "failure" to protect children dispose policymakers towards excessively rationalistic, proceduralized policy solutions that are themselves infused with anxiety and hence particular varieties of defence against anxiety? In effect, have policymakers mandated "ritualized task performance" as a solution to perceived "performance failures"? However, policy prescriptions never fully determine the implementation process, and they are always available for mediation, interpretation, and resistance on the part of organizational and professional leaders and management.

But if the form in which public policy "solutions" to profound periods of social anxiety about our capacity to protect children from harm are congruent and intersecting with the "solutions" to task-related anxiety arising from the psychic pain and anxiety of the primary task, then we are looking at an overdetermined state of affairs in which internal and external dynamics are reinforcing each other in complex ways.

Menzies Lyth and modern policy processes: from depressive to persecutory anxiety

Lees, Meyer, and Rafferty (2011) discuss the striking parallels between Menzies Lyth's typology of defensive behaviours and practices found in the hospital setting, including the secondary anxieties these defences generated, and the defensive character of policy-driven "solutions" to the succession of public and professional crises that have afflicted child care and protection work in Britain. The *Munro Review of Child Protection* (Munro, 2010, 2011a, 2011b), which aimed to dismantle the rigid, proceduralized organizational and practice culture of child protection work, may represent the most powerful example of Menzies Lyth's influence on public policy, although Munro also draws on a number of other theoretical and research traditions. However, I think there are important theoretical and practical distinctions to be articulated with respect to the origins and nature of defensive processes generated at the task and the public policy levels.

Central to Menzies Lyth's analysis is the idea that it is anxiety about potential harm to patients which drives the individual and collective need to erect defences—to offload decision-making responsibility, generate obsessional rituals around decision making, maintain emotional distance from patients, project harsh and critical voices onto junior staff, and so on. Menzies Lyth directs attention to how close contact with suffering, loss, injury, anxieties about death and dying, as well as the libidinal impulses aroused by close contact with patients' bodies, may mirror and mobilize early infantile anxiety states in staff. These core anxiety states conform mostly to what Kleinian theory denotes as "depressive anxieties", in which fears about harm done to the "other", and the consequent fear of guilt about such harm, predominate.

Lees et al. are right to point to the congruence between the varieties of defence that arise at the task level and at the public policy level, but are the underlying anxieties the same? I suggest not. Rather, the dominant anxieties inhering in, and deriving from, the public sphere concern allegations and accusations of failure, of the potential for public humiliation and scapegoating of individuals, entire organizations, and even professions, with many well-publicized real-world instances to reinforce such fears. In a performance culture, the consequences of organizational "failure" are real and rapid. Heads roll, careers are destroyed, organizations are shamed and put into "special measures", and so on. Here, the paramount anxieties concern threats to the self, not to the other, generating "persecutory anxiety", in Kleinian terms. Hence the familiar and oft-repeated observations about contemporary defensive organizational practices being directed towards "covering your back". What is implicitly lamented here is precisely the replacement of concern (albeit anxious concern) for the patient or service user, by a dominant anxiety for the survival of the professional self.

I think this is an important and useful distinction to recognize, but, of course, it is also not as neat as the above formulation suggests. First, we can see in the Menzies Lyth thesis how projections or displacements of anxiety into superiors, or onto junior staff, dynamically position them as potential "persecutors", who via processes of projective identification may then indeed enact exactly this role. In post-Kleinian clinical thought, the oscillations and dynamic interplay between persecutory and depressive states have been well theorized and illustrated (e.g., Britton, 1998). But the key point remains. Where persecutory anxiety predominates, the vulnerable or suffering other is obliterated. Where depressive anxieties predominate, there is at least the possibility of retaining emotional contact and concern for others.

So, second, when we describe policy prescriptions and the cultures of practice emanating from them as "defensive", what are we suggesting they are defending against? Is it the same kinds of anxiety that Menzies Lyth identified, or something different? It is not clear to us that the anxiety states driving policy processes are "depressive" in nature, but more that they are efforts to quell anxieties about allegations of "failure" by governments, ministerial departments, professional leaderships, and so on, as well as the political and professional repercussions of blame becoming attached to any of these. Cooper (2005b) and others (Reder & Duncan, 2004) have noted how public enquiry and media preoccupations are marked by the absence of any conscious or explicit sense of mourning or depressive reflection in relation to the tortured, dead, or severely injured children who are their supposed object of concern. Equally, these political and public processes have been emptied of any reference to the idea of tragedy or accident. Instead, a discourse of perfectability and failure or disillusion in relation to a shattered ideal predominates—"This must never be allowed to happen again, and today I am announcing measures that will ensure this."

Thus, our contention would be that when human services become the object of intense critical public scrutiny, then the likelihood is that a social dynamic will ensue that entails an escalation of generalized persecutory anxiety, organized by idealized fantasies, with accompanying defences against such anxieties which translate into an overdetermined anxiety situation at the level of front-line service provision. Cooper (2011, 2014) has conceptualized the history of child protection policy in Britain as a story of successive episodes in which the containing boundary of the formal child protection system has been breached at points of crisis, resulting in the need for some form of arbitration or "settlement" in the judicial or public sphere, before some semblance of social containment is re-established. The Francis Inquiry into Mid Staffordshire NHS Trust, successive public scandals in the wider social care domain, and the trail of crises afflicting the police service suggest that the analysis advanced here is probably applicable well beyond the particular professional case with which we are primarily concerned.

But what might all this mean for the "lived experience" of staff working within services afflicted by these complex processes, and for the vulnerable children and adults who depend on them? How have anxieties developed since Menzies Lyth's study? Given the recognition of an increasing burden of policy prescription and performance management, have persecutory anxieties replaced depressive task-related anxieties, or do the two coexist? And, in response to these, how do socially structured defences manifest and to what end? This has received less attention than it deserves, and its study requires a closer, experience-near, or ethnographic form of enquiry.

A psycho-socially informed case study

The small-scale empirical study reported here (Lees, 2014) comprised a psycho-socially informed case study. The study employed ethnographic methods of observation, interviews, and documentary analysis and was theoretically informed by the work of Menzies Lyth and by that of Cooper (2010), Hinshelwood and Skogstad (2000), Krantz (2010), and Woodhouse and Pengelly (1992). Research questions related to social workers' experiences of information sharing in the context of multi-agency working to safeguard children. Underlying the research was the recognition of the problematic nature of information sharing and a belief that it is an area of practice likely to be influenced by anxiety and defensiveness.

The cases were three social work teams within the same Local Authority Children's Services directorate. The teams were a Referral Screening Team (RST), an Initial Assessment Team (IAT), and a Longer Term Team (LTT). Practitioners in all teams were open about the anxiety-provoking and emotionally intense nature of their work, which, in many ways, is unlike any other. As one senior practitioner in the Longer Term Team expressed it:

> "You're very often taking the weight of the world on your shoulders, I mean where else, I sat back . . . one day and listened to the phone calls that were going on around me, I had one young boy of 12 that was in a sexual relationship with a family dog, I'd got another one who it was her father, and you can go round the table and you've got Mr A knocking absolute skittles of shit out of his wife, every night, night after night after night, the children are caught up in it all, you've got another baby over there that's just eaten a huge lump of cannabis and has been rushed to hospital. Where else can you actually get up, shower, come to work in the morning and it's full on?"

A great deal of anxiety and other powerful emotions such as sadness and anger were generated by the nature of these cases and by contact with vulnerable children and adults. Powerful emotions in many forms were present in the workplace, and we agree with Paul Hoggett (2014) that anxiety is not the only emotion that needs defending against. Social workers often reported using humour, for example, as an antidote to the sad and upsetting nature of the cases they dealt with. Social workers also spoke about dreading visits with particular service users and of being threatened and even physically attacked. This was not unexpected terrain—such issues have received attention within the academic literature (e.g., Ferguson, 2005; Taylor, Beckett, & McKeigue, 2008; Waterhouse & McGhee, 2009). These powerful emotional states resonate with the primitive anxieties aroused within nurses in pursuit of the caring task in Menzies Lyth's study.

Perhaps somewhat surprisingly, then, given the nature of the cases described above by the senior practitioner, most day-to-day worry and anxiety for social work practitioners within the research site was caused by the demands of heavy workloads and competing priorities, within contexts of high demand and scarce resources.

> "You're kind of almost always catching up with yourself and you're almost always doing just enough. Which is why they get into this cycle of case open, little bit of signposting, case closed, referral, case opened, signposting, you know. You just kind of get into the circle. And time and time again you see families coming round and round and round ... I think that's probably the worst part, is that if the caseloads were lower and the timescales weren't so prominent I think we'd all do a much better job than what we do, even though we all do the best we can with the time we've got." *Social worker, Initial Assessment Team*

Reflecting the increasingly "informational" nature of social work (Parton, 2008), it now appears that "managerial" anxieties are inherent in the working lives of social workers, as much as exposure to abuse, distress, and hostile clients. Menzies Lyth identified a number of these "managerial"-type anxieties in her study, but she described them as being secondary consequences of the adoption of socially structured defences against the primary, primitive anxieties of the nursing task. For example, she suggested that fears about operational breakdown (or inability to cope with the work) resulted from the defensive adoption of rigid and inflexible processes. Frustrations about the lack of opportunity to use professional judgement was described as another secondary anxiety of this rigid organization of work. In this study however, it is clear that external pressures of high demand for services and policy blueprints for work organization have given these anxieties a life of their own. They bear down on social work teams from outside and are as powerful, if not more so, on a day-to-day basis than anxieties about caring for vulnerable children.

Reflecting this, I have suggested that the political and policy context of twenty-first-century organizations was likely to have created a new set of anxieties, related to the prevailing conditions of market economy (see chapter 3) . These I named as:

» Rationing anxiety (relating to the scarcity of resources).

» Performance anxiety (relating to performance management and audit).

» Partnership anxiety (working in networks and multi-agency arrangements over which no one has central control).

Anxieties expressed by participants across the three teams strongly resonated with the broad categories defined above. "Rationing" anxieties commonly expressed included staff and service cuts, pay freezes, staff turnover, and outdated/unsuitable office space. "Performance" anxieties related to heavy workloads, high administrative burden, competing priorities, performance management, and being able to do work well enough in pressured environments exacerbated by cases that are ambiguous and complex. While social workers' concerns about their own ability to function well and to keep children safe were depressive in nature, persecutory anxieties abounded as well. These related, in particular, to the monitoring by senior managers of social workers' adherence to case timescales. While social workers often did not feel this to be a fair reflection of the work they were doing, they were nevertheless susceptible to feelings of shame when they were flagged as falling behind.

> "When we get work allocated to us that's late, day one starts on the day of the referral regardless of when it's allocated to us. So we all have periods of time where all of our initial assessments are red because they're over 10 days, so then you're like, I'm crap, I don't do my job . . . So you then do the monitoring report avoidance: I'm not looking at it because I know I haven't done it so you don't need to remind me every day." *Social worker, Initial Assessment Team.*

For social workers within the Longer Term Team, the court environment added a tranche of anxieties about their ability to present evidence that was clear enough to stand up to cross-examination and to allow the best judgements to be made for children. In such adversarial environments, persecutory anxieties did not seem to be misplaced.

> "Especially when you're in court, you're going to have to give evidence in court, court proceedings are a bit of a blood bath. You get cross-examined, you need to be very thorough in your work . . ." *Social worker, Longer Term Team*

"Partnership" anxieties were often forcefully expressed and related to the lack of willingness by some other agencies to engage fully with the child protection process, with social workers feeling that they were sometimes literally, as well as figuratively, left "holding the baby".

Socially structured defences against anxiety

How, then, did defences manifest in response to the anxieties outlined above? In this study, socially structured defences were taken to be working processes that appeared to be disproportionate responses to the situations encountered (Trevithick, 2011) and that were linked to secondary consequences such as delays, frustration, and despondency. These were identified tentatively by the researcher during observations and checked out in interview with research participants. As a result of this process, a new socially structured defence was identified, which took the form of "spotlight" practice to clarify and justify the focus of professional attention in the context of limitless demands, under-resourcing, complex cases, and rigid performance management. This took a variety of forms, in particular attempts to make sure that overworked teams were doing the right work in the first place (manifest in boundary and threshold disputes), to make facts and proposed courses of action as explicit and clear as possible, and to rehearse and repeatedly check actions and decisions to ensure that mistakes are not made.

Boundary disputes between agencies and the careful checking of referrals by social workers has previously been identified as a defensive feature of practice related to heavy workloads (Broadhurst et al., 2010) and feelings of being under siege (Woodhouse & Pengelly, 1992). Within the research site, boundary disputes were most evident at the internal boundary between the Referral Screening Team and the Initial Assessment Team. Despite the existence of a detailed local authority threshold document within the research site, interactions between the two teams were characterized by disputes over the nature of cases and whether they warranted social services intervention. Within the IAT, there was criticism of the RST's ability to filter cases "correctly". The IAT would sometimes immediately close cases that had been referred to them by the RST, or send them back with requests for further information. In turn, there was a perception amongst the RST that their decisions were being scrutinized and unfairly criticized by the IAT. Within both these teams, there was also frequent criticism of the inability of some other agencies to make appropriate, or detailed-enough, referrals. As the team leader of the IAT explained, the careful manning of in-boundaries represented a defence against taking on the "wrong" work when they already have too much of the "right" work to do. If this happens, nothing can be carried out to a high-enough standard.

> "If we took that premise we'd be inundated and we're already too busy as it is. So if we are doing all the wrong work we can't get to the right work . . . I'm like 'STOP! Don't do anything!' because we have a principle here that we must challenge this. We have to challenge this, because if we

> start taking things . . . I think has been part of our problem why we've been so inundated, because we can't just be a 'yes' team."

Prominent in the Longer Term Team, elaborate processes for clarifying and checking facts and decisions had developed. Social workers' tasks were often laid out, and reported back, on a step-by-step basis—with seniors setting out specific tasks for social workers to complete; the latter would then complete the task and return straight away to the senior to feed back. Involvement of a number of levels of management in discussions about casework were also frequently observed. Practitioners described multi-layered systems for the approval or sign-off of documentation—in particular, court paperwork. While the involvement of seniors/team manager in the day-to-day details of cases was perceived as supportive by some more junior members of staff in need of reassurance, it could cause frustration for those with more experience, who identified associated consequences of delay and role overlap.

> "Why is that system in place that 3 people need to check it? I don't understand, isn't someone competent enough to be able to check that report once, sign it and send it off? Because otherwise it's making the whole process even longer than what it needs to be, because ideally you'd want your court work done a week before. It's impossible." *Social worker, Longer Term Team*

These defences resonated with a number of those identified by Menzies Lyth regarding decision making and checking with seniors; they also had an obsessional aspect to them, as Halton suggests. Taken together, they represented socially structured defences against anxieties about carrying out important and risky work in contexts characterized by lack of time, resource, complexity, and ambiguity, but importantly also in the shadow of an omnipresent inspectorial "management system in the mind" that was not the sole product of task-related anxieties or defences against these.

Spotlighting was used to shed light on complex and ambiguous cases, to illuminate decision making, and to sift out any of the "wrong" work. While a spotlight is good for illuminating the details of dark and murky contexts, it is less able to provide a wider view, and therein lies the problem for inter-agency information sharing and collaboration. Important issues may be lost in the shadows outside the concentrated, but narrowly focused, spotlight of professional attention. Information that is lost in the shadows cannot be shared. To allow a more diffused view to be taken, there is a need for enhanced "holding" of professionals through an increased sense of role clarity and containment within the organizational and inter-organizational contexts.

The professional "self" and modern organizational anxieties

My own experience of intensive post-qualifying training work with social workers and health care staff strongly suggests that the state of affairs we are describing has profound impacts on the lived experience of the workforce at all levels. Most people enter human service work with a primary, if sometimes naïve, desire to "help others", to provide care, and to engage humanely with complex human predicaments. Whatever else their roles and task demand, they want to be able to work in a relationship-based fashion and to use their professional self as a central resource in doing the work. Menzies Lyth's great contribution was to show us how complex and disturbing this simple aspiration actually transpires to be, as we encounter the reality of suffering, injury, mental pain, internal and relational conflict, fears of death and dying, and strong libidinal impulses in both others and ourselves in the ordinary course of such work. However, the hopeful dimension of her work was to show that if organizational boundary conditions are attuned to these realities, allowing space for continual non-judgemental reflection upon working experience, then the satisfactions and rewards of the work may far exceed any detrimental impact of the anxieties it generates.

Equally, the hopeful dimension to the case study described above is that *despite* carrying the weight of persecutory and depressive anxieties, practitioners nevertheless expressed much joy and satisfaction in their work with their service users. The respondent below surprised the researcher with this comment—as most of the conversations they had shared in the office were to do with his stress concerning the magnitude of his workload and performance-management reports.

> "...We all are, I think, making some difference somewhere, some positive impact somewhere. Um you know, not all the clients would be happy with us in terms of like the parents or dads and mums, um, but I think we are working for the children. They may not even be able kind of, share their views when it's really like um, you know a teeny tiny child, um, but I, I am glad I'm doing it and I feel good by the end of the day. Most of the days (*laughs*). Not all the days, most of the days! I feel good that at least, you know, we have done something about that situation, about the child."

Thus, in the research process, Amanda Lees was arguably subject to something analogous to a negative transference from her subjects. Given an opportunity for open-ended narrative disclosure, it is the weight of frustration, anger, and despair that is first communicated to a receptive listener, because these feelings and thoughts have no proper organizational outlet. This is a frequent experience for psychoanalytically attuned researchers, and it facilitates access to the complexities and subtleties of the lived experience of subjects, much as a good organizational consultancy would aim to do. The thinking and research advanced in this chapter suggests that negative, externally generated "boundary conditions" have become much more prominent in shaping the context of service delivery, and that the anxieties and defences involved typically invade organizational "space" and, beyond this, the mental space that is the self of the worker. An account of lived organizational and personal experience by a child protection worker, written some years ago now and also quoted in chapter 11 of this book, illustrates this vividly:

> I am working in a factory. I have been working there for the last five years. When I started working there I did not think it was a factory. It didn't look like a factory, not from the outside and not from the inside. . . .
>
> The management measures (in percentages) the reports of initial and core assessments completed on time, and compare these to other teams. When the team manager reports these statistics in team meetings, I can recognise how my body becomes tense and my heart rate increases, and I get very angry. . . . I have voiced my resentment to this ritual but it was ignored by managers and other colleagues. [Cooper, 2009, pp. 174–175]

My experience of receiving experienced, well-qualified practitioners—like the one who wrote those passages—into post-qualifying "continuing professional development" trainings is that they are often, in effect, depressed by their working lives. However, they do not usually know this, but gradual exposure to both the experience of reflective "work-discussion" spaces (Rustin & Bradley, 2008) and also experientially inclined seminars on contemporary policy processes enables them to begin to feel and know about their depression and the frustration and anger that underlies it, and to rediscover a "lost" or buried sense of professional vocation rooted in the desire to engage with other people—a professional self that has gone into hiding. But crucially, *both* forms of training experience are required. Reflective case discussion that does not engage with the baleful impact of the organizational and policy environment goes only so far. Recognizing, naming, and recovering some sense of personal agency in relation to the different, intersecting, and frequently congruent forms and sources of anxiety delineated in this chapter—those that are located primarily in the difficult nature of the primary task, and those that flow from the organizational, managerial, and policy environment—becomes possible and, to a degree, liberating.

Fear and dread: a contemporary "structure of feeling"

In a much-cited but not very well developed or articulated passage, Raymond Williams introduced the idea of a "structure of feeling" to suggest that particular social epochs or formations are characterized by pervasive, organized, but not cognitively very "legible" collective emotional experiences. A structure of feeling, he writes,

> . . . is as firm and definite as "structure" suggests, yet it is based in the deepest and often least tangible elements of our experience. It is a way of responding to a particular world which in practice is not felt as one way among others—a conscious "way"—but is, in experience, the only way possible. Its means, its elements, are not propositions or techniques; they are embodied, related feelings. In the same sense, it is accessible to others—not by formal argument or by professional skills, on their own, but by direct experience . . . [Williams, 1993, p. 18]

Menzies Lyth's seminal thesis about the functioning of social systems as a defence against anxiety captured something of the same idea, but at the more specific, micro-level of organizational culture. The sense so many people have of finding in her work the articulation of something they have "always known", but for which they have had no language or concepts with which to make sense, attests to its potency. For example, recently I encountered a senior professional and psychotherapist who had been my social work tutee twenty years ago. She recalled, "I told you about my struggles in the agency where I was on placement. You said, 'Go and read Menzies Lyth'. I did and I never looked back."

The practitioner in Amanda Lees's study who described "taking the weight of the world on your shoulders" was referencing the astonishing variety, complexity, and emotional intensity of his team's encounters with individual suffering, family conflict, infantile vulnerability, and adult perversion and neglect—the demands of the primary task. The practitioner who expostulates, "Why is that system in place that 3 people need to check it? I don't understand, isn't someone competent enough to be able to check that report once, sign it and send it off?" is referencing something different that, in our view, cannot be fully explained or understood with the conceptual resources Menzies Lyth bequeathed to us.

Today, alongside the three core forms of "externally generated" anxiety afflicting organizations discussed in chapter 3 and above, we must include a further one: survival anxiety (see Figure 4.1). The particular form this takes in modern British child protection work has been the main subject of this chapter, a fear of catastrophic failure arising from "missing something" and becoming the locus of blame for the death or serious injury of a child. Some people do not survive the consequences of being so blamed (Shoesmith, 2016), whether they were in any true sense responsible for the "failure" or not. This especially virulent form of organizational anxiety is, in fact, just an extreme instance of a more general preoccupation with "organizational failure" that permeates our society and which was explored in depth in Cooper

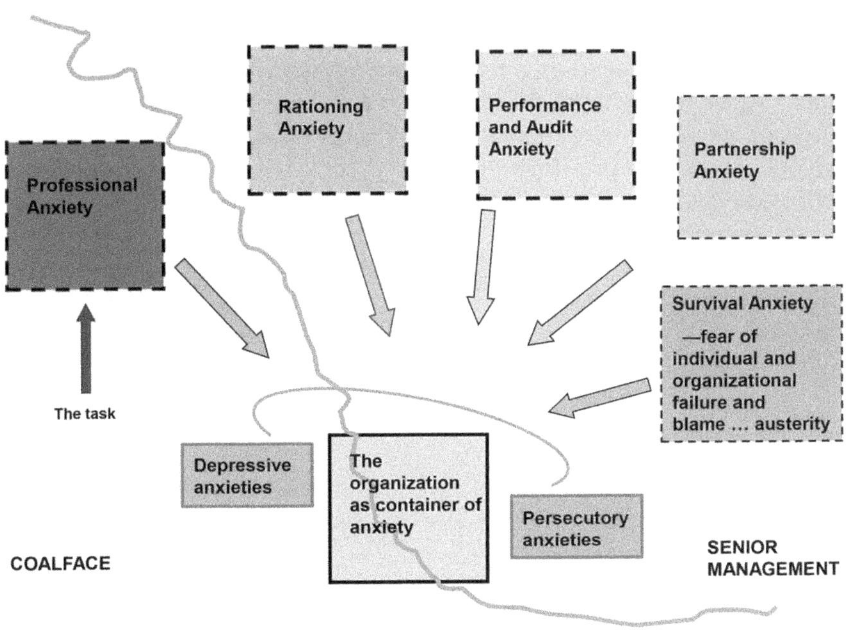

FIGURE 4.1. The accumulation of modern organizational anxieties, showing the tendency for these to evolve from a predominantly "depressive" to a "persecutory" form.

and Lousada (2005). In the post–financial-crash climate of modern Britain, economically grounded fears of organizational collapse are acute and seemingly also chronic, and they mingle in a diffuse fashion with the more psycho-socially rooted threats to survival discussed in this chapter. However, they coalesce into a single pervasive experience, namely fear for survival of the professional self in its organizational context. Figure 4.1 is an attempt to capture this story in diagrammatic form.

It is in the nature of defences, whether functional or dysfunctional (and most defences are sometimes or in part one and sometimes the other), that they successfully disguise or obscure the threats, feeling states, and fantasies to which they are an attempted solution. As a paradigm instance of good psychoanalytic work, Menzies Lyth's research allows us to see beyond certain kinds of apparent bureaucratic mindlessness to the literally "dreadful" sources of anxiety located in the task that generate defensive practices. There is much further work to be done in order to provide corresponding empirical support for the proposition that the pervasive obsessionality of modern managerialist practice arises, in part at least, from a collective need to defend against equally pervasive fears of personal and organizational failure emanating from, and situated in, a public sphere organized by a competitive, risk-averse policy and political climate. The sociology of modern organizational development suggests many forces other than just task anxiety at work in producing the total picture we are describing, forces imbued with but not simply reducible to processes of projected anxiety or social ambivalence. In line with Raymond Williams's observations, we can only undertake this more fully psycho-social enquiry via a rigorous engagement with the experiences of social subjects inhabiting the live world of such psycho-social formations, and in these terms the work reported in this chapter is a beginning.

CHAPTER FIVE

Talk talk: what is the "Tavistock Model"?

Mental health—hard labour

In this chapter, I offer an account of the "Tavistock Model" of clinical thinking, training, and organizational life. This "model" is much quoted, debated, and contested but much less written about or defined. It provokes polarized responses. Some people love it and some detest it, but probably more are baffled when called upon to describe it, even if implicitly they understand it well. I hope what I set out here helps clarify and illuminate matters, but equally I hope it provokes further debate and argument because, as I suggest, the model itself concerns the nature and value of open thinking and open-mindedness, not closure and dogma.

The chapter is written from a particular point of view that informs most of the chapters in this book, the particular blend of thinking that a social worker and psychoanalytic psychotherapist brings to the world of mental health work and to clinical practice generally. Really, there is not one "Tavistock Model" because each professional discipline draws on its core theoretical and methodological preoccupations in contributing to and constructing the total institutional model of thinking and practice, so the idea of a family of models is perhaps a more accurate way of describing the situation.

Stability or closure of our identities is an illusion. Too much change and transformation is intolerable. We seek closure as a refuge from the anxiety and mental turmoil it creates in us, and we do this via the stories we tell about ourselves and others. These narratives structure our world, supported by and giving shape to powerful conscious and unconscious feeling states. But the stability of these emotional structures is illusory. They protect us at the same time as they limit our possibilities and our freedom of thought and action. This is not a new paradox, but for individuals and organizations—especially those devoted to alleviating mental suffering—it is given fresh significance by the times in which we live. The political, intellectual, and policy culture we inhabit ceaselessly demands innovation, transformation, and renewal. Thus it promotes one side of the paradox and demotes the other, the necessity of illusions, the need for a place to rest and think.

Developed capitalist societies are traversing rapid and turbulent change following the economic crisis of 2008–2009, and the theories, practices, and organizations that have embodied their efforts to tackle social suffering, inequality, and mental pain in society for the last fifty years are subject to radical questioning. In such times, some have argued that conservatism is a form of radicalism—the struggle to preserve progressive and humane social and organizational practices in the face of "modernization" becomes paramount. But how do mental health services distinguish between unhelpful resistance to change and the struggle to conserve a valuable and valued endeavour?

Here I explore how the Tavistock tradition might help our understanding and handling of some of these contemporary dilemmas. These questions are not "just theoretical"—emotional and social suffering is real, immediate, and damaging for those afflicted. The model of mind and social life sketched out in this chapter as an answer to these questions is not simple, but arguably its validity has stood the test of time. It is not simple partly because, as the philosopher Jacques Derrida (1988) said, "If things were simple, word would have gotten around." The paradoxes outlined above are part of the complexity, but they are often played out in an oppositional manner, as arguments involving entrenched positions taken by competing schools of thought and practice that could be supporting one another.

Historically, this is true within the Tavistock itself, and so this chapter attempts to model something that we all tend to preach but often find hard to practise—tolerance of difference, ambiguity, tension, or contradiction—in search of an integration of ideas. Broadly, this chapter suggests that the two main schools of therapy that the Tavistock houses—family systems and psychoanalysis—tend to occupy different sides of the paradoxical coin, with family systems favouring a narrative of openness and fluidity, and psychoanalysis one of marginal stability and closure. But the difference between them may, on closer inspection, transpire to be credit-card thin, their argument with one another a case study in what Freud (1930a) called "The narcissism of minor differences". If this idea has validity, then it is transferable to many other instances of tension and conflict in contemporary organizational, social, and personal life.

Tavistock "philosophy" proposes that the best way to surmount entrenched states of hostility, conflict, intransigence, misunderstanding, or impasse is to put people in a room together and talk—anywhere between two and a hundred and two, as we shall see. Eventually, if things go well, some new version of the fixed, troublesome "truth" will emerge. This notion of knowledge or truth as a *process* of engagement, a dialogue leading to discovery, echoes the now rather unfashionable tradition of dialectical thought and philosophy.

In common with many mental health service organizations, the Tavistock Clinic enterprise is a human project that tries to engage with some of the most profound, intractable, and painful realities facing us all. It is not "above and beyond" these realities, but entangled with them, and thus as vulnerable to their insidious and damaging aspects as are the people it tries to help. This chapter suggests that what unifies its different schools of therapy and practice is a commitment to direct engagement with lived human realities, in search of imaginative transformations that release people from incarcerating social and psychological pain and relationships. On this view, a potential for change and transformation is at the heart of what it means to be "mentally healthy", but so too, it turns out, is a capacity for stubbornness—"knowing your own mind" and what you stand for (and will not stand for) personally and organizationally. The quest for that which, to paraphrase Shakespeare, "alters not when it alteration finds" is the heart of the matter. But in a period when change is visited on us by forces that seem beyond our control, the problem of how to navigate our personal and organizational identities *with integrity* becomes acute.

But if individuals and organizations dedicated to such helping practices are themselves subject to the same forces that act upon and within people seeking help, then the former must continually work to release themselves from the grip of self-incarceration, and this necessitates a dialectical movement between openness and closure. The tendency for psychotherapeutic practitioners and institutions to assume an omniscient and inferiorizing stance towards the suffering or afflicted "other" is evidence of the absence of such movement.

The dedication of experienced mental health practitioners to continuing rigorous supervision and self-analysis signals its presence. The psychic and organizational strain of sustaining the continually self-questioning stance necessary for openness and transformation speaks to the contemporary requirement for "vulnerability" in our psychological stance as professionals (Hirschhorn, 1997) and the likely impossibility of sustaining a mental posture of perpetual "negative capability" (Bion, 1970, p. 43; Keats, 1817). Whatever you call it—reflexivity, self-awareness, deconstruction—staying "mentally healthy" is hard mental labour.

A bottom line?

The notion of an "enterprise" speaks to the fact that the work of the Tavistock, like that of most contemporary organizations, is not confined inside its geographically located organizational boundary (Cooper & Dartington, 2004). The enterprise is an "open system". It is the set of total exchange processes transacted among a wide range of cultural, professional, social, psychological, spatial, and temporal elements (the intersecting and overlapping relationships and movements among patients, trainees, professionals, public, the media) that constitutes the whole. Does this depiction reflect actual changes in organizational structure and form—a trend towards a more dispersed or networked form of organization with less well bounded spatio-temporal coordinates—or just a new way of seeing what has always been the case, a release from the *illusion* of well-bounded institutions with a clear, single primary task? Or perhaps a complex blend of both in which new ways of seeing enable different ways of being, and *vice versa*?

These questions haunt most modern organizations, as well as many key social institutions like political parties. They also sound very like the questions people ask of psychotherapy itself—(how) can simple talk give rise to change, and have I really changed or just altered my view of myself, freed myself from constricting self-representations? However, there are important "realities" that are in tension with any view of organizations as somehow liberated from the straitjacket of tradition and modernity, free to impose themselves on the high seas of the market if only they have the self-belief to pursue a project of domination.

The financial crisis of 2008–2009 brought this home—money turns out not to grow on trees, even if temporarily it proved possible to persuade ourselves that it does. Ultimately the "bubble" burst because "sub-prime" home owners from poor American communities *could not pay* (Lanchester, 2010). There transpired to be a "material" constraint on endless growth. Likewise, the Tavistock Centre building in Swiss Cottage, and other physical sites it now "owns", are obstinately there, housing expensive staff whose salaries consume most of the organization's budget, using heat and light that must be paid for. But by whom, why, and what for? If psychotherapy and organizational consultancy can make us a little freer we should welcome this, but we also should not confuse freedom with immortality or omnipotence. Buildings crumble, water pipes burst, bodies age—we die, or find that our credit has reached its limit, and no amount of "thinking it differently" can alter certain brute facts.

This chapter describes some of the invisible "technologies" that occupy the space between despair in the face of life's struggles and brute facts, and the possibility of finding hope and meaning. They concern ways of engaging in personal, group, organizational, and social *development* evolved at the Tavistock over many decades, practised and refined every day by many thousands of people who have learned from them. These "methods" are directed at creating conditions for seeing and experiencing the self, relationships, family, and social relations *differently*. Thus, they are about liberating imaginative and imagined futures from the imprisoning hold that unconscious beliefs and emotions, languages and scripts, and restrictive or oppressive social and organizational practices can exert.

So, what are these "technologies"? After ninety years of Tavistock history, do they remain relevant to others in modern times? Are they evolving or static? Is there still hope for the vision of mind and social life they embody?

The Observer

A child psychiatrist and family therapist who worked at the Tavistock Clinic for over thirty years was fond of saying, "You can observe the Tavistock's core technology any time you want to. Just walk down Fitzjohn's Avenue and look through the windows of the seminar rooms. What do you see? You see groups of people sitting in a circle, talking, thinking together."

He is right. But what are these people talking and thinking about? How can such a seemingly mundane and passive activity generate so much passion, commitment, and controversy? If there is anything in this method, can it be described, explained, made transparent, or is it a form of mystique as its critics and detractors often claim? Reviewing the first phase of a large consultancy intervention, I asked the CEO who had commissioned the intervention what the feedback was like. "Positive from a lot of people" he said. "And the others?" I asked. "In short, same old Tavi bollocks", he replied.

My approach to the writing of this chapter is deeply rooted in my own experience of working at the Tavistock as a teacher, clinician, manager, and consultant, but also as a learner and student. It is therefore necessarily personal, partial, and selective, but also questioning and critical. I have loved working and learning at the Tavistock. It has shaped my life in many respects. But this does not prevent me thinking, sometimes several times a day, "Aarrgh . . . Same old Tavi bollocks".

The observer peering through the windows of the Tavistock is engaged in the very same "Tavistock" activity that so divides people's responses to this institution. He is looking, reflecting, wondering, formulating an idea and a concept for what he sees, thinking about an experience. Central to this is an awareness of his own mental processes, which are focused on other people and what they might be up to. He is interested in "other minds" as well as his own. And so he is engaged in a relationship. Out of such simple but actually quite sophisticated mental activity is born the possibility of being a person with a mind and of something called "society"—a system of relationships.

One, several, many, one, . . . ?

There is not a single Tavistock Model and method. As will become clear, there is in reality something more akin to an extended family or constellation of ideas and practices, linked by a set of family resemblances. But how close is this family? Traditionally, the institution has thought of itself as housing two main clinical and theoretical paradigms—systemic family therapy and object-relations psychoanalysis—although much of what the Tavistock is known for is extensions, ramifications, and applications of these originating practices. In recent years, in response to shifting public and professional demands and forces in the mental health field, other clinical traditions such as Cognitive Behavioural Therapy (CBT) and Mindfulness have found a foothold, and new models of short-term dynamic psychotherapy are being developed and tested. So far, it is unclear how this more inclusive trend will affect, or be affected by, the core methodological tradition. Change processes in individuals, couples, families, groups, and organizations are central to what the Tavistock Clinic and its services are all about, and, as the wider world changes, so must the institution itself.

But how does change occur? And what makes up the more stable or perhaps "stuck" identity of the person or system of people which is endeavouring to change? Are there limits to the possibility of change, and if so what are they? Investigating these questions will direct us to the heart of what Tavistock models and methods are about and reveal that although there is not a single or final answer, perhaps there is a deep structure, a relatively stable pattern, to the set of fundamental human predicaments (and ideas about these predicaments) with which the methods and models try to engage. Practitioners of psychoanalytic therapy and family systems therapy are more or less united on one thing: a certain kind of talk or conversation is essential to the possibility of change. This is why the people you can see through the windows of the seminar rooms could be teachers and learners within either, or indeed both, traditions.

However, an investigation of the physical spaces within which Tavistock clinical practice occurs tells a different story. I once saw a family for assessment in the Adolescent Department psychoanalytic family therapy service. The young man who was the "index patient" walked into the room with his parents and immediately turned to me in alarm. "What's that?" he asked, pointing to one wall of the room. I think he half knew what it was. The wall was shuttered, and behind the shutter is a one-way screen. Beyond the screen is a second room where, if this had been systemic family therapy, one or more clinicians—the reflecting team—would also have been sitting with the shutter open, so that they could observe the family while remaining invisible to that family. This scene can represent the point of departure for an important thread of the inquiry of this chapter. When we observe human behaviour and interaction as therapists, what are we attending to in our search for understanding of their pain and suffering? When we talk, what kinds of "insight" is our talk based on? As clinicians, can we successfully observe ourselves, without the help of others?

The two dominant traditions of psychotherapy at the heart of Tavistock practice transpire continually to divide, reunite, divide and reunite again around answers to these questions. This pattern of division and reunification may be the closest we can come to a "consensus" about Tavistock models and methods. The situation is perhaps analogous to that which faces theoretical physicists following the discovery of quantum mechanics. The deepest structure of physical reality seems to be a fluid and unpredictable contradiction, but it supports something—everyday physical reality—that appears stable and in many ways predictable. If comparison between the Tavistock tradition and the greatest achievements of modern science smacks of arrogance, perhaps this is a clue to the fiercely divided responses that the institution attracts, and also the continual emotional turbulence that is a feature of its daily working life. Adherents of the Tavistock's models and methods believe they really know something important. To others, it can seem like dogma, a faith in obscure and arcane rituals that have little foundation in observable reality.

"Stop that fucking thinking!"

Whichever main tradition of practice and theory someone subscribes to, they might agree about one thing. The experience of being observed by others can feel intensely threatening. Perhaps this worry lay behind the reaction of the young man mentioned above on seeing the shuttered screen. I was introduced to this thought in my first hours of work at the Tavistock. I went to a meeting room and found two senior psychoanalysts there. I introduced myself, whereupon one of them declared, "It's a terribly difficult place to work, because everyone is scanning the unconscious the whole time!" "I'm not", responded her colleague. "Of course you are", said the first, "You must be. You're a psychoanalyst!" Whichever of these one takes to be nearer the norm, the presence of so many figures inside the institution who are *believed* to be scrutinizing each other may explain why, on entering the organization, perfectly well-balanced people often experience an acute discomfort that is also hard to pinpoint.

Students on trainings who undertake planned observations of infants at home, or of organizational settings, frequently encounter unexpected resistance to the idea of "being observed". The reason is that the observer is often experienced as an intensely critical, judgemental presence, rather than the interested, dispassionate one they believe themselves to be. Being observed, and thought about, can feel very exposing, as though someone is "looking with x-ray eyes" into the murkiest and most shameful parts of the mind. Ronald Britton, a psychoanalyst who worked at the Tavistock for many years, has given much thought to the question of how and why some people develop to be so terrified of their own minds that they cannot think about themselves, while others are much more at ease. He relates this to the nature of the relationship between the parental figures a person carries inside him/herself. If someone has a sense of parents who get together in a friendly way to think about the person, then internal "mental space" can get established, a capacity to encompass feelings and thoughts about the self and others in a relatively free and easy way. But if the internal figures are felt to be too hostile or critical, ganging up against the child, then mental space closes down and the observing figures must be fought off. Britton describes working with a patient who he believed found his private efforts to "commune with himself" about her very threatening, and she burst out with "Stop that fucking thinking!" (Britton, 1989, p. 88)

Talk, experience, and "reality"

Psychoanalytic and systemic practice are united in questioning and interrogating the "surface" or taken-for-granted dimensions of how people represent themselves and their relationships in their talk. But they conceive of this project in somewhat different ways. A psychoanalytic therapist had been seeing a woman twice weekly for a number of years. She found the patient consistently "difficult"—hostile, spiky, cryptic, unreflective—and often felt on the back foot, as though the patient were permanently at war with her, and was winning. The patient often complained that the therapist wanted to impose her own theory or account of matters and did not take seriously the patient's own account of her troubles and their origins. Clearly she did not feel "understood". The therapist acknowledged to herself and her supervisor that, unusually for her, she did not feel she easily recognized or identified with the patient. She felt her psychoanalytic work was rooted in many years of personal therapy, during which she had encountered in herself fragments or vestiges of most states of mind her patients presented to her. But this woman had always seemed different, and the therapist often felt she was failing the patient.

One of the patient's complaints was that the therapist wilfully ignored her belief that her emotionally isolated childhood had been blighted by "lack of social contacts", an absence of friendships. The therapist did, indeed, consistently probe other ways of understanding the patient's childhood, and adult, isolation. But these efforts always resulted in a "rupture" between the therapeutic couple.

Then one night, after several years of this work, the therapist had a dream involving the patient. She described it as the most lucid dream she had ever had about her analytic work. In the dream, *she returned to her childhood home for a weekend to meet some friends and go for a walk. But she had also invited the patient to accompany her. On arriving at the house she became worried about leaving the patient alone there while she met her friends, and she wondered whether she should not forgo the walk and keep her patient company. This is what she did, after rendezvousing with her friends and explaining*. The dream prompted the therapist to remember how isolated her own childhood had been in many ways, and how anxiously attached to her own mother she remembered becoming. On one occasion, the therapist's mother had gone away for the day and had arranged for her daughter to travel by herself to visit a favourite aunt. But the young therapist had been frightened, feigned illness, and stayed at home with her father.

The therapist spoke of this experience in psychoanalytically familiar terms: she described how in the dream the patient was clearly "a part of herself", the anxious, isolated child she thought she had long ago left behind. Her decision to stay at home and keep company with the patient, forgoing the pleasures of "social contact", both echoed the patient's talk of her own childhood and reminded the therapist of how anxious she herself had once been. Much to her surprise, since she believed herself to be a "well-analysed" therapist and fully conscious of her own childhood loneliness, she now believed that she had long been in a defended state with respect to this patient's own painfully withdrawn and isolated experiences.

Perhaps this vignette crystallizes something of how psychoanalysis "thinks" and also helps explain how psychoanalytic work is done, as well as why it can feel so threatening. In psychoanalysis, there is always a quest to look within or beyond a representation—in words or images—for signs of other representations, layers of psychic "reality", that infuse one another with meaning and feeling. The assumption is that these representational layers connect with one another, although not necessarily in a fixed or permanent way. Indeed, psychoanalytic work may be dedicated to revealing such connections in order to allow them to de-couple. Fixed, layered ways of thinking and feeling about the self and relationships may be at the root of the mental pain or symptomatology that first brings a person, family, or couple to therapy. Once disclosed, the faculties of the conscious mind can observe these layers of connectedness and reassess them. This is a way of restating some of Freud's original formulations about psychoanalysis and how our minds work. "Free association" was the means of revealing the unexpected but meaningful series of connections, and the concept of the "primary process" contained his account of the "laws" of unconscious thought processes that generate them.

But how do we know whether this account is right? What justifies the assumption that different representational layers of thinking and experience connect in a particular way? Are there not deep and unexamined assumptions at work here about what lies "beyond" or "behind" manifest experience or surface talk, whether of dreams or other registers of experience. In fact, the therapist's assumption that the patient stands for "a part of herself" in the dream is a deeply "theory-laden" proposition. Her "story" about the dream is just that—a story—and, moreover, exactly the kind of story that a psychoanalytic therapist *would* tell under such circumstances, because the stories they tell are scripted according to assumptions of just this sort.

Suddenly it looks as though psychoanalysis can be hoisted on its own petard, its own discourses vulnerable to the same unexamined and fixed beliefs about how things are connected that it purports to be so good at disclosing in the thinking of others. Moreover, experience would suggest that were the therapist to narrate the dream a second time, the narrative would be subtly different and probably suggestive of new or differently nuanced interpretations or thinking. Or, because they usually cannot resist doing so, other psychoanalytic therapists hearing or reading this "story" will want to add, "But it could also mean . . .". Which is the "true" or valid narration, and where lies our access to any core or "real meaning" as distinct from its various possible narrations? If there is a "reality" beyond the range of stories we can tell about an experience, access to it seems to be denied by the slipperiness of the same portal—language—that promises us entry to "the real". Under these circumstances, philosophical integrity surely demands that we focus attention on what can be more certainly grasped, namely how people talk, narrate, tell stories about themselves and their relationships. In this way of thinking about "talk" and its connections to mind and relationships, we have crossed over to the kind of talk that systemic therapists favour as their starting point.

Once this shift of focus has been achieved, difficult questions about whether there is or is not anything "beyond" talk may just dissipate. Perhaps there is such a realm, but what we can now assert is that experience, relationships, states of mind—everything that is the proper object of a concerned therapist or mental health professional—is also "constructed" through language and story-telling. If painful and disabling states of mind or relationship can be produced in this way, they can also be "deconstructed" through therapeutic work that encourages us not just to "tell it like it is", but to "tell it differently". Transformational conversations, rather than a search for "truth", become the watchword.

Narratives of difference, similarity, resemblance, . . .

Given these areas of convergence and divergence, how similarly or differently do therapists of different persuasions such as psychoanalytic and systemic actually work, and conceptualize such work? And do the practices themselves provide further clues to the nature of the elusive unity-in-diversity of the Tavistock's models? These are large questions, and I will confine myself here to one important dimension of the answer which may signal a further "conjunction of differences". Both schools of therapy are committed to a view that the work cannot be done without a live, here-and-now, self-conscious entanglement of the therapist in the process of the work. Systemic therapists call this reflexivity, and psychoanalytic practitioners call it working with the transference and countertransference. Each entails its own idea of self-observation.

When a family or couple meets the systemic therapist(s) who, classically, will be supported by the presence of a reflecting team or colleague, the meeting is conceived as a joining of one system to another. This joining occurs through the medium of communication—not only talk, but also other visible and describable communications: who sits where in the room, who opens the narration, who supports the terms of the dominant narrative, and who might be dissenting from it through silence, and so on. The therapists in turn are invited to "join" this communicative pattern in particular ways and not to disrupt or question it in others. Their contributions cannot but confirm or disconfirm particular patterns or scripts. There is no "neutral" communicative stance, only an evolving co-production of new here-and-now patterns that will reinforce certain constructs in the "client system" and/or disturb and perhaps re-frame others.

Somewhere in this web of communicative patterns and silences, or told and untold storylines, lie the sources of, and possible solutions to, whatever difficulties have brought the system to therapy. As the therapists become "positioned" within the developing conversation, their observing faculty—colleagues positioned out of sight behind the screen, but in contact with the process—may intervene to propose adjustments to the therapists' conversational strategies with respect to those of the family. This is talk about talk about talk, and the account you are reading is talk about talk about talk about talk; if you were now to discuss this with your friend then it would be talk about talk about talk about talk about talk.

Part of the aim of therapeutic intervention in this modality of work might be to encourage the articulation of previously unheard, or unvoiced, "lines of narrative". The children may never have heard the parents speak of their own childhood difficulties; the parents may never have heard a child's account of his experience of the parents' arguments; everyone may have been silent since mother's miscarriage, or father's redundancy. In systemic therapy, a central aim is to keep the narratives moving, developing, shifting, open.

As this process unfolds, an observing psychoanalytic therapist would be engaged by, and interested in, aspects of the total experience that the systems therapists seem to focus on less. For example, if a parent immediately engages one of the therapists, or one of the children, in a critical and disparaging manner, the psychoanalytic interest is likely to focus on the powerful feelings involved in the exchange and what this may mean in terms of projective processes within the family. If the therapist suddenly feels small, useless, and unable to speak for fear of provoking another attack or creating an argument, she may speculate that this provides insight into how anxieties associated with dependency or insecurity are managed in the family; people are not just silenced from talk about such matters by particular communicative strategies, they are also made to *feel* small and stupid by those who find these very subjective states too hard to bear for themselves. Feeling like this can be very close to believing it to be true. In this way, the structure or patterning of the "system" becomes deeply inscribed in individual subjectivities as well as residing in interpersonal relationships that continually reinforce and re-produce these more private states of mind.

From here, the psychoanalytic inquiry may begin to follow similar lines to those outlined above with respect to the therapist's dream. What deeply inscribed emotional experience and beliefs about being a child does the parent import into this family from his or her own experience of being parented? In other words, what is the *internal* grandparental and great-grandparental "system" inhabiting this family in the here-and-now? Disclosing the continuing presence and influence of these absent or long-dead figures, the family ghosts, may become an important focus of therapy. Enabling family members to speak of these formative experiences and memories constitutes psychoanalytic story-telling.

Feet on the ground or head in the clouds? Reflexivity and countertransference

As the psychoanalytic therapist consults herself about her own immediate experience of feeling attacked and disparaged, she tries to sort out its meaning. Is this a communication, via projection, of how a child typically comes to feel in this family when the parent reacts to feeling threatened? Is it how the parent experiences his own internal parental figures? Is it about the contemporary anxiety of starting therapy? Is the therapist herself especially sensitive to critical attacks of this kind? Or maybe all of these?

In systemic theory and practice, there is, as we have seen, a trend towards the interminable re-framing of narratives via meta-perspectives on each narrative layer. In psychoanalytic thinking, there is an equivalent trend towards infinity in the search for both lateral and biographical associations of meaning and feeling. On the face of it, one appears to direct attention outwards and one inwards, the former linking systemic theory to the work of holistic philosophers like Gregory Bateson and Spinoza, and the latter to traditions of mysticism, an association explicitly invoked by one of the most prominent psychoanalytic ghosts walking the corridors of the Tavistock: Wilfred Bion. Reflexivity can be described as the discipline of thinking about thinking and talking about talk so as to constantly interrogate and locate one's own position within a system; attention to the countertransference can be described as the discipline of continually scrutinizing the subjective states aroused in the therapist in order to locate evidence for one's position within the field of unconscious mental activity generated by the therapy. Both are central to the working practices of the Tavistock, and both signal an important paradox or tension about the institution's position within the contemporary cultural and social field.

Does the centre hold?

So, do therapists of either (or, indeed, any) persuasion occupy a privileged position with respect to their *knowledge* of the individuals, families, or organizations they encounter and try to work with? I have represented both systemic and psychoanalytic practice as constituted by a kind of radical scepticism, and yet the institution of the Tavistock is often portrayed as a centre of dogmatism. We live in an everyday world increasingly defined by professed ideologies of choice and relativism, a "post-traditional" and "post-hierarchical" world in which "difference" and multiplicity of perspective replace unity or dependence on received authority—sometimes as descriptions of how things *are*, sometimes of how they *should* be, or sometimes both. Psychoanalytic and systemic thought have played a part in bringing this world into being. In different ways, both have contributed to "de-centring" the knowing subject from a privileged position with respect to itself and others. The necessary immersion or entanglement of the therapist with the psychic and systemic life of the "patient", and the correlative need to be permanently engaged in freeing or locating oneself, is one index of this.

Yet both schools would wish to defend their respective contributions to modern mental health work as solid, even necessary, to the possibility of good practice. People who come to the Tavistock to learn often say that that they quickly feel themselves to be better grounded, more confident of their own position in relation to the intense emotional and intellectual complexities of their work. On the other hand, at the heart of the "Tavistock bollocks" lobby's complaint is a frustration with a perceived reluctance to just get "stuck in" rather than engage in ceaseless reflection. To ask that we reconcile these positions might be to fall prey to the very desire for unity and cohesion, the search for a master narrative, that I have suggested is antithetical to the spirit of Tavistock thought. Is this the final paradox? Perhaps, perhaps not . . .

A method for the madness

How do these various interlocking principles of therapy translate to the domain of teaching and learning? Writing about the practice of "Work Discussion", one of the central pedagogic Tavistock methods, Sebastian Kraemer (2011) says:

> Someone presents material from his or her work followed by comments from others. The facilitator holds back to allow students to engage with one another, to experience rivalry, to experiment with authority and take risks with their imagination. "What did it feel like to listen to this case? How do we understand these differences in perspective?" Silences are tolerated. Every contribution is regarded by the facilitator as presenting different but equally valid aspects of the case or theme. [p. 95]

Again, we notice the theme of "participatory democracy", now threaded through the therapeutic learning process. In her discussion of this method, Margaret Rustin writes that:

> The aim is to strive for a relatively theory-free and non-judgemental attitude to everyone involved, including oneself. The apparently meaningless is just as valuable in the record as the probably or obviously significant. The debt to the free-association method in psychoanalysis is an obvious one. [M. E. Rustin, 2008, p. 11]

The approach is also much informed by Bion's concept of "containment", or "container–contained", perhaps *the* most revered (and important) of psychoanalytic ideas in Tavistock discourse.

Given much of what has been said in the preceding pages, it might seem that we could characterize the entire Tavistock project as one of "containment", an institutional effort to create conditions in which "unthinkable" experiences in the minds and relationships of patients, professionals, organizations, and citizens can be rendered "thinkable" and speakable. In the psychoanalytic paradigm, the struggle is *towards* representability and language. In the systemic, it is rather more *with* the representations and forms of speech or language we already have.

Inability to represent and verbalize emotional experience can be disabling, imprisoning, a form of traumatic mutism; the discourses we do create are sometimes liberating and sometimes constraining, oppressive, and often both. Discourse *is* closure, and closure generally excludes or "others" one or another group or individual. The *experience* of authentically "free-associative" psychoanalytic work is that you never tell it the same twice over. Instability of "representation" is the norm. A fundamental precept of systemic work is that this is how it ought to be, if conditions for growth, change, development, and the realization of transformational possibilities are to be sustained. Psychoanalysis is good at showing us how unconscious processes and defences—splitting and projection—generate closed or compartmentalized psychic structures and systems. Systems thinking is good at disclosing the discursive strategies and formations that constitute the (micro-, meso-, macro-) social embodiment of these. Spaces of hope, rather than of despair, are dependent upon the contributions of both to producing cultures of liquidity.

The start of the world

Is there a Tavistock practice where these world views meet and exchange notes? The answer is perhaps yes and no. The tradition of group relations work *should* be a main site of rapprochement, and is perhaps becoming so. The tension concerns how psychoanalytic and systems practitioners understand "systems" and work with them. The latter tend, perhaps, to see the former as having appropriated their systemic territory in a naïve psychoanalytic manner, while the former find difficult the tendency of the latter to ignore "unconscious process". Nevertheless, alongside work discussion, it is group relations events that are probably the most original Tavistock contribution to the study of "ordinary madness". Lasting anywhere between 3 and 14 days, with between 25 and 100 members, the central learning task of these events is to "study" the experience and process of the various small and large groups that constitute the whole "temporary institution". Group relations events bring into being a small, complex society, a full-blown "psychodynamic system".

To be part of the first minutes of a group relations event is rather like being present at the origin of the universe itself, or the birth of a child. First, nothing; then something, and then awareness of this something—and finally perhaps a name for it is spoken. But this can be harder than it sounds. At the start of one such conference, the hundred or so members were invited to gather in the large room available for "whole-system events", together with the conference staff, a number of whom positioned themselves at the edges of the space. The task was to form into groups of eight and select a member of staff as facilitator, thus forming the "small study groups" that would meet throughout the life of the conference. No guidance was offered about *how* to achieve this objective, except that it must be done in silence.

As people circulate silently around the room, small knots begin to form—pairs, threes, fours. They know they must eventually coagulate into groups of eight. A group of four meets one of three, and they decide to join. Lacking a final member, they look about themselves. Small groups that have not become attached search for possible partners. In less than half a minute, only a very few individuals have not attached to someone else. Groups of nine or ten are now obliged to silently negotiate about who might leave them and search for another home. The first groups of eight begin to "dock" with group leaders positioned at the edges of the room. Somehow, after a few minutes a dozen groups of eight people and twelve group leaders are linked to one other. They begin to leave the room to begin the first of their small study-group sessions.

Taking up the task of the conference, one small group begins to reflect upon the experience of its own formation. Members speak about the anxiety—terror, even—of finding themselves isolated and homeless. Some pairs and threes describe how they had instantaneously clung to one another on the basis of prior familiarity. Others say that all other members of the small group are unknown to them. The group starts to reflect on the mysterious process by which they selected their leader, and one member says that she tried to guide the group towards him because "he looked friendly", which perhaps signals the depth of the underlying fears already aroused. In his turn, the group leader is thinking about what he is hearing, as well as his own experience of group formation. After a few minutes he intervenes and says that two thoughts occur to him to help make sense of this: "survival" and "any port in a storm . . .".

These events are the experiential counterparts of philosophical ideas developed within other traditions, recalling, for example, Martin Heidegger's existentialist notion that each of us is "thrown" into the world and struggles ever after to live authentically with the terror of this condition, which is not of our choosing. The scientist and philosopher Jesper Hoffmeyer starts his book *Signs of Meaning in the Universe* (1996) by speculating about the evidence for material ripples or "scar tissue" left over from the Big Bang when the first "lumps in the universe" formed, producing the differentiation that is the necessary precondition of meaning and eventually communication.

The opening phases of the above conference replicate this chaotic, turbulent process of something—human groups—forming irrevocably out of the homogeneous soup of the totality. But they also speak to the unconscious terrors that lurk beneath the everyday ebb and flow of organizational and social life: the intimacy of strangers, the fear of abandonment and isolation, the ubiquitous propensity for inter-group rivalry, hatred, and cooperation.

An alternative space: The Democratic Republic of Swiss Cottage

So, do not be seduced or persuaded by the apparent calm, the *very thoughtful* atmosphere you might detect as you peer through the windows on Fitzjohn's Avenue. This is just an important outward display masking an equally important inner turbulence and turmoil. At their point of contact, as we have seen, is talk, language, and some other processes that inform talk both from "within" and from "without" in order (this is the hope) to generate meaning, understanding, and change.

In order to enter the main building of the Tavistock, you are obliged to step through a glass doorway, turn right for a few paces, go through another glass door, and then turn left. This peculiar arrangement has survived a recent refurbishment of the whole entrance lobby. Occasionally one can observe perplexed first- time visitors to the building twisting and turning as they try to fathom the way through. It is hard to think of another modern public building with a more convoluted boundary-crossing point. On the other hand, the Tavistock is one of the least "securitized" of public spaces—no passes, no signing in and out, and not much CCTV. All day, from 7.30 in the morning until well past 9 in the evening, there is a constant flow of people in and out, sidestepping one another in the glass of the entrance—staff, patients, students, visiting teachers, guests, conference participants. Unless you are very familiar with the day-to-day activity of the institution, it is nearly impossible to identify who among these people belongs to which group, and in different ways a high proportion can lay claim to several of these identities.

The corridors of the clinical directorates in the building suggest a different story. Sequestered, noiseless (the rooms are excellently sound-proofed), anonymous except for tiny brass nameplates, the lines of uniform brown wooden doors are normally closed. Occasionally, one of them will reveal an open-plan office space, but more typically they house the clinical, teaching, managerial, and administrative staff, with many rooms trebling up as office, clinical, and teaching space. At first sight, it seems anyone can stroll into the Tavistock and wander its mostly uniform spaces, as though it were an oversized, misplaced public library or art gallery—there are modern paintings hanging on almost every available wall space. But from time to time you will catch sight of two or more people making their way towards one of the offices, silently, awkwardly—therapist and patient (or maybe family or group) arriving for (psychoanalytic) therapy. What happens between them behind the closed door, in the sound-proofed room, is intensely private and strictly "out of bounds" to anyone else. You can gain easy access to the Tavistock for many purposes, but equally many of its core activities and spaces are tightly patrolled. The position of the sliding Vacant/Engaged sign on each door is a key signifier of the continually oscillating transitional space between openness and closure, private and public, inner and outer worlds, that the Tavistock exists to study and engage with.

The creative tension—and synergy—between the necessarily privatized space of the therapeutic setting and the location of the

Tavistock within the NHS and public sector was for many decades embodied in its unique internal structure of management and decision making: hierarchical, tribal, paternalist, on the one hand; democratic, fluid, complex, and subversive, on the other. Until the system was abolished by the Board of the newly formed "Foundation Trust" in 2005, the clinical staff of the organization elected all its own managers for fixed-term periods of office. These practices were understood as extensions of the models of mind, and psychotherapy, found at work behind the closed doors of the many corridors. Therapy is a process of helping people to recover agency and *authority* for the living of their own lives. Authority of any kind cannot be simply claimed or asserted or "supposed"; it must be found, discovered, conferred. Within a group, it must be *both* granted and accepted or "taken up". This kind of democracy and authority is both elective, but also—continually—participatory, because leaders and followers are in permanent relationship with each other.

But once again, do not be seduced, however admirable, appealing, and progressive this model of organizational life may seem. Under the surface of democratic "maturity" and sophisticated notions of authority, naked urges for power and domination continued to lurk. In recent years, more than one medical consultant has been heard to voice the idea that doctors are in truth *primus inter pares*—first among equals—among the professions, thereby doubly enraging colleagues with an assertion of superiority cloaked in arcane language. Some exponents of some Tavistock clinical orientations have subtly abandoned courtesy and "participation" in favour of arrogant stances towards patients and students. Perhaps all clinical groupings and many individuals are guilty of such regressive behaviour at least some of the time. But each instance that affects a patient, student, or member of the community damages the Tavistock, providing ammunition for those who wish to attack its reputation and self-idealizations.

But, for many, the strong conviction persists that the loss of this 75-year-long tradition of therapeutic republicanism may have marked a decisive shift in the Tavistock's fortunes in the modern world. The boardroom battle that decided its fate was nasty, brutish, and short. Within the managerialist climate of the modern NHS, under the scrutiny of the ominously titled "Monitor" which oversees the governance and performance of Foundation Trusts, it was almost certainly unrealistic to hope that a democratic model of management could survive. Better then to kill it first, rather than face its extermination by an outside force? These are the decisions any "organizational ego" must confront in assessing its relationship to "external realities".

Democracy is one of the organizing principles of all "therapeutic communities", a tradition of residential "milieu" psychotherapy, with which the work of the Tavistock has much in common. Therapeutic provision of this kind has had a hard time in the NHS in recent years, and it may be dying out within the British public sector. Therapeutic democracy is subversive, challenging the norms and practices of mainstream psychiatry and mental health practice, research, theory, and ideology. Uneasily positioned within mainstream NHS structures and its modern instruments of "governance", and so often seen by those who do not know or understand its practices as a centre of traditional elitism, the Tavistock's claim to radical status is often disputed. To those who do know it, and have worked or learned there, its claim to represent a true alternative is not much in question. In a period of managerialist conformity, however, its capacity for long-term survival as a true "Other" is facing new challenges.

Through the decades, the Tavistock has negotiated many challenges to its future. If such challenges ceased, this would surely signal that it had already lost its institutional potency. Its core purpose is to disturb "the order of things", and of language, in pursuit of such freedom from everyday personal and social suffering as can be attained. Perhaps this is the lot of all organizations dedicated to improving mental health. Our society is deeply ambivalent about the mental pain it causes people and suffers in return, and it responds with equal ambivalence to those institutions that aim to engage and work with this pain. Tavistock theories and methods offer some hope that all of this turbulence can be made at least "thinkable" and thereby rendered a bit less toxic and destructive.

Since this chapter was first written, external conditions for the NHS and the public sector generally have significantly deteriorated. The "survival anxieties" induced as a result, and discussed more fully in chapter 4 of this book, afflict the Tavistock as much as any organization. My own experience is that this is producing adverse internal organizational conditions and a greater sense of internal threat to the survival of the "model", as though the "same old Tavi bollocks" state of mind has taken up residence inside the institution as a kind of saboteur. The saboteur state of mind represents the overwhelming fear that if we do not "get real", then we may not survive, and getting real means detaching from an unquestioning commitment to the preservation of aspects of the model because, quite simply, they may not any longer be affordable. But really this is just the latest twist in the unceasingly anxious process of negotiating between the pleasure principle and the reality principle—what we would wish things to be, on the one hand, and what external realities such as balancing the financial books tell us are the ugly facts of the matter, on the other.

We can never "bound free" once and for all from the unconscious, language or society, so the project is a never-ending struggle. We cannot live without "closures", but every settled state, equilibrium, unexamined assumption, or habit of organizational mind that helps constitute the creative "authority" of an institution is also the basis for possible corruption, oppression, and ultimately death. An organization whose purpose is transformational must be prepared for and capable of self-transformation.

CHAPTER SIX

Institutional racism: can our organizations change?

The ordinary and the extraordinary

Over two decades ago, in 1987, the Tavistock Clinic, the intercultural psychotherapy centre Nafsiyat, and the University College London Department of Psychotherapy collaborated on a series of intercultural psychotherapy seminars. The papers arising from these seminars are full of incisive, forthright, and even courageous theoretical and clinical discussion. I quote from the introduction to the collection:

> The "whiteness" of the Tavistock, the host institution, both representative and symbol of psychoanalytic psychotherapy within the NHS, was frequently pointed to in the context of this provision. The arguments for and against the Tavistock as a white, privileged institution were well-voiced. A point also made was that here was re-enactment of the characteristic intercultural psychotherapy—the "insider" Tavistock being equated with the white therapist, resources at hand, and "outsider" Nafsiyat with the black, disadvantaged patient (University College to be located in the middle). [Ingham & Fitzgerald, 1988, p. 1]

When I arrived to work at the Tavistock Clinic in 1996, my guess is that in terms of its "whiteness" and its capacity to confront the meaning of this, the institution had not changed at all in the intervening decade.

My mother used to make a delicious hot pudding comprising a suety dark-chocolate base covered by a layer of pale, creamy meringue. It was called, without irony I fear, "South African pudding". Early in my time at the Tavistock, I often used to think of this as an apt-enough metaphor for the social structure of this organization. It was not in fact a "white" organization. But without exception, I think, all of the so-called senior staff—the tenured clinicians—were white, while the administrative staff were significantly black, Asian, or mixed heritage, and the lowliest "support staff" almost entirely so. I experienced this as shocking. Not primarily because I experienced the situation as morally or politically reprehensible, but because of the contrast with the institution I had just left after ten years. This was an outer-London social work training department based in an Institute of Higher Education recently incorporated into an old university. In this department, a significant majority of students were black or Asian, and the teaching staff group comprised roughly half black and Asian members and half white. Through the 1980s and early 1990s, it seemed to me that London became steadily more ethnically diverse and multi-racial, as did the profession of social work. Against this background, my working context in the same period seemed just ordinary, and my new working environment at the Tavistock Clinic nothing short of extraordinary.

Today, this is no longer true. There has been real and meaningful change at the Tavistock, especially in the ethnic diversity of the student and trainee population, and the provision of training programmes and conference series dedicated to, for example, black leadership and African psychology. No doubt some of the change would have occurred "organically" without the focused, and funded, effort that I and other colleagues led over a period of years starting in about 2000. But interestingly, the notion that change *should* be "organic" was one form that I believe institutional resistance to change assumed. Much like patients in therapy, people did not particularly like being challenged or "confronted" (however gently and thoughtfully) to consider change. A common response to our explicit project to stimulate change was that "really, it needs to happen 'organically'". This chapter takes it for granted that institutional racism is a variety of organizational defence. Do we expect our patients' defences to simply dissolve in the face of reasoned argument? I suspect not. Organizational change is painful, and those attempting to lead change must expect to suffer a bit.

In more recent years the British Association of Psychotherapists (BAP), now incorporated into the British Psychotherapy Foundation (BPF), also embarked on a targeted development project around race, equity, and access to its trainings. The Tavistock is a public body, part of the NHS,[1] and as such has been subject to more stringent equalities legislation and monitoring regimes in recent years than most independent sector or charitable institutions. This has helped legitimate the Race and Equity initiative in the organization, but equally it has provided no guarantee of authentic development or change. The BAP/BPF relies heavily on voluntary rather than paid effort for the strength of its organizational culture, and this creates a different set of organizational conditions and dynamics for internal change processes.

Enclaves

Institutional racism is both a manifestation of organizational resistance to change and a main source of that resistance. But tackling institutional racism is about the pursuit of ordinariness, about creating conditions wherein, at a minimum, organizations fully reflect the ordinariness of a multi-ethnic society. The fact of multi-culturalism, or the fact of ethnic diversity in our cities, does not mean that racism has been eradicated in our country, but it is evidence of ordinary, hopefully irreversible social change. The fact that within such multi-ethnic environments one can find organizational enclaves apparently almost untouched by these changes is surely evidence of something deeper and more troubling. Almost without exception, I suggest, the major institutions of psychoanalytic psychotherapy and psychotherapy training in this country are just such enclaves. I know less about other psychotherapeutic modalities, and I cannot speak for them.

Thus, in certain sectors of modern British society, there is a sense that we have already moved beyond the familiar binary thinking that organizes questions about "white institutions" and an excluded "black or Asian" population. Today, many younger ethnic minority people no longer identify in a simple way with these categories; people of dual heritage, or multiple ethnic origin, and, indeed, people of white Anglo-Saxon origin who grew up and went to school in communities of complex ethnic diversity, have a correspondingly complex and nuanced view of race, of race relations, and of the many shapes and forms that racism can adopt. The shifting requirement to negotiate hybrid identities at both a personal and a social level is their starting point in lived experience. On this view, there is no longer a simple white majority or a simple excluded, marginalized, and denigrated ethnic "other". Black or Asian people may well occupy positions of power, prestige, or seniority in organizations, political associations, and community contexts. Old barriers have come down, and if this does not imply that racism has disappeared, it no longer conforms to the models developed by anti-racist activists in the latter part of the twentieth century.

My proposition, however, is that this kind of development in the direction of more fluid and complex race relations has largely not yet penetrated the major institutions of psychotherapy in this country. The capacity to evolve such complexity depends not primarily on acts of imagination, theoretical sophistication, or private clinical inquiry, but on people of diverse origins with different experiences and histories of the painfulness of race relations *living, working, and actively engaging with one another* around these questions. It is a matter of active, and often uncomfortable, dialogue across the lines of diversity. This is not yet really happening, because it can't—our psychotherapy institutes are not internally homogeneous on many indices, but on certain important ones to do with race they are. They still are white institutions. In his paper "Against the Celebration of Diversity", Farhad Dalal develops this idea of engagement:

> . . . in speaking I, of necessity, negate something of the Other. The response of the Other in some way negates the negation, and my response negates that, and so on. This movement is transformative as it is conflictual. And it is transformative for therapists and patients alike. It is this kind of process I would call engagement, in which the self is risked and, as it is risked, it moves, shifts, and changes. [Dalal, 2008, p. 18]

Where Dalal speaks of the self taking risks and changing, I would merely add "and institutions". In posing these matters as starkly as I am, I do not wish or intend to arouse guilt and anxiety. As Dalal also observes:

> The fact that our profession suffers from these issues is no different from any other human grouping. It cannot be otherwise; the predicament is born of the human condition, and so we are all bound to be embroiled in similar processes. The fact that as a profession we live in a glass house should not necessarily prevent us from throwing stones at other glass houses, as long as we are also able to accept and reflect on similar communications. [Dalal, 2008, p. 14]

But are we able to accept and reflect on our institutional life in this way? Are we able to act in pursuit of organizational change in this respect? I want to propose that there are some rather general conditions of organizational life in this country that make it very hard to do so; but I want to spend more time examining a number of phenomena that I believe are rather particular to the culture of psychotherapy institutes, that obstruct our capacity to engage with this most difficult of questions: are we institutionally racist?

20–60–20

During his campaign to promote change in the Metropolitan Police Force in the wake of the Macpherson Report's findings about institutional racism, the Metropolitan Police Commissioner Sir Ian Blair observed that when you embark on this kind of project you can reckon that about 20% of the workforce is behind you, about 20% dead against you, while the remaining 60% are biding their time, watching and waiting to see which way the cookie of change starts to crumble. To me, this rather rough-and-ready analysis seemed intuitively accurate. We should remind ourselves that he is describing the situation facing leaders who try to promote change in what we can loosely describe as "white" organizations, those with a preponderance of white staff, which constitute the vast majority in this country. In effect, Blair is saying, "A sizeable minority of people are actively or latently hostile to the project of opening up our institutions so that black, Asian, and other ethnic minorities may enter them and have hope of advancement within them on fair and equal terms; but more worrying, perhaps, a sizeable majority don't really care one way or the other." Clearly, leading this kind of change in almost any organization is destined to be a lonely business.

Organizations differ—this, of course, goes without saying. Perhaps every organization is in fact unique. But from the perspective of race relations and ethnic composition, there are specific "structural" factors—broader patterns in social life—that bear upon the situation facing different categories of organization. What kinds of people are in a position to seek entry into professional organizations depends upon the availability of a "pool" of suitably qualified and experienced potential applicants within any group, and in this country it is only in the last couple of decades that we have achieved a situation in which there is such a pool of black, Asian, and other ethnic-minority people qualified and experienced and, other things being equal (which I shall go on to argue they are not), *eager* to enter our institutes of psychotherapy training. The impact of such "structural" factors on entry to professional training arenas was clearly visible in the social work department in which I worked.

We offered two kinds of entry to training: non-graduate entry, leading to a professional social work qualification with a Diploma in Higher Education, and graduate entry leading to the same professional qualification but with a Master's degree. Over 10 years, the ethnic composition of these courses did not shift a great deal. On the undergraduate entry programme, about 50–60% of students were black and Asian; on the graduate entry programme, it was around 20%. These figures were consistent with other programmes in metropolitan areas across the country. In the last ten years, this situation has changed, and the Tavistock Clinic in collaboration with the University of East London now runs a graduate-entry social work qualifying programme on which the black and Asian student intake is normally a majority. In the 1970s and 1980s, there was a familiar political analysis of institutional and other varieties of racism that explicitly, and often exclusively, linked these processes to class structures. Class position was, and of course arguably still is, strongly associated with educational achievement and opportunity, and in that period the predicaments of most black Afro-Caribbean and many Asian people in this country could be legitimately explained as an aspect of class location. With the advent of mass higher education, there is now a much more fluid state of affairs.

At the threshold

I often ask myself, "How many of these young black, Asian, and Asian and African social workers at the Tavistock, trained in a modestly rigorous psychoanalytically informed manner, will in the end find their way to the profession of psychotherapy, and successfully complete a training?" From experience, the omens are not so encouraging—at the Tavistock Clinic, over the years there were a number of black and Asian trainees who completed the long and very demanding adult psychoanalytic psychotherapy training. Almost none of them moved on to become members of the senior staff group, while a steady flow of white trainees always did find their way back into the institution, or on completion of their training sought and were offered posts within (what we ambiguously refer to as) "the establishment". At the BAP, a very small percentage of the (much larger) adult psychotherapist membership are visibly members of an ethnic minority, but just below the surface of the organization's public discourse there are many (as yet not very systematically verified) tales of those who dropped out, were refused entry on grounds that bear the hallmark of prejudice and thoughtlessness, or who did complete their training but also have a tale to tell. I shall return to this later, but surfacing these stories was one part of the BAP's initiative to explore the roots and the dynamics of what some members were at least brave enough to think, and say, might be the problem of institutional racism.

To sum up briefly at this point: There is, and long has been, a tradition of psychoanalytic clinicians engaging incisively, thoughtfully, and openly with questions of racism in the consulting room, and with what psychoanalysis can offer to the wider project of understanding and combating racism of many kinds. This is important and necessary work, but by itself it manifestly does not impact much on the organizational dynamics and resistances that are my central theme. The historical paucity of black and ethnic-minority entrants to our training institutes is partly a reflection of wider social structural factors governing race and opportunity in our society. But there is more, and we need the courage to face that "more". I have mentioned these other considerations, because there is actually a need to set them aside in the project of deepening our understanding and engagement with this problem. Not to cease acting upon them, but to cease allowing ourselves to be diverted and distracted by them as we raise the much more uncomfortable question (to paraphrase Farhad Dalal) about what sort of light passes into our own glasshouses, what is filtered out without us even noticing, and how, and why?

In various ways, then—structurally, culturally, psychically—perhaps we stand at the threshold of change while black and Asian people stand, mostly, on the other side of our doors. Why? I suggest that they may be waiting for us to do something about the situation inside our glasshouses. If anyone wants to characterize this as passivity or even hostility on their part, I want to turn that thought around and say it speaks, rather, to our need to exercise leadership—leadership, quite literally, to put our houses in order.

Secrecy and special knowledge

Why might a profession dedicated to understanding and transforming difficult, conflictual, subtle, painful, perplexing, and resistant forms of human experience be blind in the face of social relations of similar quality? I want to propose several kinds of answer. First, it is the very fact of *social* relations that presents itself as an obstacle. The psychoanalyst Wilfred Bion once wrote:

> It is important to recognize that that there is a world in which it is impossible to see what a psycho-analyst can see, although it may be

> possible for some of those who come for analysis to realize that we see certain things which the rest of the world doesn't see. We are investigating the unknown which may not oblige us by conforming to behaviour within the grasp of our feeble mentalities . . . We may be dealing with things which are so slight as to be virtually imperceptible, but which are so real that they could destroy us almost without our being aware of it. [Bion, 1994, pp. 319–320]

Whether you consider this to be a statement of supreme confidence in what psychoanalysis offers to the world, or one of extraordinary arrogance, I think it captures something vital about what psychoanalytic institutions *believe* themselves to be the guardians of—a very special kind of knowledge, made more so by the fact of its "virtual imperceptibility", and the consequent difficulty (though not impossibility) of exposing to scientific investigation the means by which this knowledge (of unconscious processes) is generated. Michael Rustin has captured something vital about the significance of all this when he characterizes psychoanalytic institutions as a variety of "secret society". He refers to

> . . . the requirement that the analytic relationship be segregated from everyday life, so that the transference of the analysand (and in more recent psychoanalytic thinking the counter-transference of the analyst) be enabled to develop in the segregated setting of the analytic relationship, without the impediment of circumstantial knowledge of the daily reality of the analyst's life and character . . . While other professionals might wish to keep their non-professional lives or even their other professional activities distant from any particular client . . . in other cases this does not seem to be a *technical* requirement of their work. [M. J. Rustin, 1991b, p. 95, emphasis in original]

Rustin goes on to describe two different institutional forms in which psychoanalysis is propagated—the British Psychoanalytical Society and the Tavistock Clinic—both of them constrained by this tendency towards organized professional "secrecy", but with the former tending more towards social closure (carrying the risk of social conservatism as a result) and the latter more towards social accessibility (entailing the risk of diluting the "essence" of analytic goals and methods). The problem he concludes,

> . . . is to combine these two forms of analytic activity: that devoted to maintaining the standard and purity of the fundamental analytic work, and that which seeks to extend its scope and social influence. [M. J. Rustin, 1991b, p. 113]

I want to extend these observations in a rather obvious way. All psychoanalytic organizations are surely divided *internally* by this tension. Perhaps every individual psychoanalytic clinician is thus divided, wherever she may position herself, or be located by others, on a spectrum running from pure investigator of unconscious process to proselyte of the social significance of psychoanalysis. Some psychoanalytic clinicians and theorists hold that the unconscious is itself a socially generated phenomenon; some hold that it necessarily precedes the "entry" of the individual into social relations and always remains elusively beyond the grasp or control of the social subject. But I think Freud's central discovery was that unconscious life is—or in psychopathology is—a kind of closed universe with its own self-generating creative and destructive powers. Probably all psychoanalytic clinicians have encountered patients, or even aspects of themselves, where the mystery is how so much mental suffering can seemingly ensue from so *little* in the way of external causes.

Here I want to introduce a simple empirical observation in support of the hypothesis I am advancing. The Tavistock Clinic is a complicated place, where the psychoanalytic psychotherapeutic project takes many forms in terms of clinical work, research, and training. I think those parts of the institution most dedicated to something approaching the pure or classical practice of psychoanalytic psychotherapy have progressed the most slowly in opening themselves to the multiracial world in which they are located. Conversely, those disciplines and units who practise and train for psychotherapeutic work in less strictly clinically controlled conditions have made bigger strides in this respect. This situation is ripe for splitting, with clinical and theoretical "purists" squaring up to social and political "traitors", all of which has uncomfortable echoes of the very problem we are trying to tackle: the tendency in racialized or racist thinking and practice to see "difference" as a murderous threat to a phantasized purity of identity, and to construct rigid defences against invasion, incursion, and ultimately intercourse with the feared "other".

The problem of tolerance

The second cultural obstacle I want to discuss concerns tolerance, and "thoughtfulness". A colleague of mine is fond of asking, "What is the technology on which the Tavistock depends?" The answer, he says, can be seen if you walk along Fitzjohn's Avenue and look through the windows of the seminar rooms. What you will see, most hours of the day, are groups of people sitting in a circle, talking. They are thinking together, being "thoughtful". This is what psychotherapists are good at—being thoughtful about painful, perplexing, difficult matters associated with mental pain. Setting aside questions of race, culture, or racism for the moment, the matters we spend our time being thoughtful about often concern relationships of domination, control, exclusion, and so on. We may be mainly focused on the manifestations of such relationships in the inner world of patients—how, for example, emotional neediness and dependency is ruthlessly attacked and excluded from conscious awareness, isolating the subject from the possibility of believing that ordinary nurturing relationships based on vulnerability are something that can be risked. We are likely to be examining how such internal relational scenes are played out in a living manner in the transference–countertransference dyad of therapist and patient. Our deep conviction is that if these living, dynamic, emotionally charged relationships can be understood, emotionally contained, and processed by therapists, then there is a chance of modifying the destructive work they do in patients' lives and minds.

In essence, as therapists we try to tolerate emotionally what it seems patients find intolerable in themselves. We try not to retaliate, blame, capitulate, or by other means *enact* a role in these relational scenes, though we are alert constantly to the pressure we feel in ourselves to do just this. Indeed, it is from this pressure that we gather our most important data about patients, and their habitual, usually unconscious, ways of relating to themselves and others. We may sometimes feel that a patient is using the opportunity of therapy to be a complete bastard to someone—us—but in the consulting room we refrain from ever putting it quite like this.

Hyper-alert to the dangers of enactment, I think that as a profession we easily confound this with the idea that action of any kind is dangerous. A while ago, after I had helped secure some funding for two posts dedicated to a race and equity initiative at the Tavistock Clinic, I was discussing their role with my boss at the time, a man I deeply admired and respected. I referred to the idea that these posts would contribute to a process of change in the institution. "We don't want them to help us change," he snapped at me, "we want them to help us think."

The "materiality" of institutional racism

The culture of liberal tolerance has many dimensions, and many I believe we should profoundly respect. But I am not alone in arguing that it contains deep-seated contradictions. These include the idea that at some level "we are all the same", all "human". Of course, who could not subscribe to this notion in some sense or other? But liberal tolerance *uses* this idea defensively in my view, by focusing on "diversity" or "difference", and, as Farhad Dalal (2008) observes, "The thorny issues of power relations are forgotten in the miasma of celebration (of diversity)" (p. 12). Or, as I have heard it put very recently in the context of trying to discuss institutional racism in a psychotherapy institute, "The important thing is to accept that we are all racist". Again, one might hardly take issue with this. The defensiveness is in the way that these statements "flatten" our stance towards the *particular* manifestations of racism that are alive in the here-and-now—of this discussion, of this interaction, in this institution, at this period in its history.

Now again, rather curiously, we all accept that we do not think about our patients (or indeed ourselves) in this way as psychotherapists. We do not interpret the patient's communications or read our own countertransference as an illustration of some universal and abstract expression of human nature. It may be this, but the process of insight, change, transformation in therapy proceeds from engagement in the here-and-now with what is alive, active, in the encounter between patient and therapist. Understanding a patient, or ourselves, cannot proceed via some process of logical deduction from universals; it always proceeds, or at least begins, inductively from an engagement with particulars. "Particulars" ultimately do not stand in opposition to generalities or universals; they partake of them, but in unique ways that have to be discovered anew each time.

So, as one engages with an organization in a project of examining its possible institutional racism, a frequent response is, "Why this kind of racism, why do you focus only on black people/Irish people/and so on?" The answer is always the same in my view: the right focus is the actual problem that presents itself, if we can bear to know it as a problem. It may be that, for example, Jewish members of an institution *are* experiencing discrimination or racism, as well as black or Asian people. If so, then the particular form this takes is a legitimate focus of thought and action. But if there is no *living* experience of something in the here-and-now that is affecting people—despite whatever terrible histories of oppression people may carry inside them—then there probably is not, as it were, a condition to treat. In the old Marxist language of the social sciences I learned as a young person, this is called the "materiality" of social relations. What is material are particular, living, embedded varieties of social relationships.

The "internal racist" and the institution

What happens when an organization does attempt to engage with itself around this sort of agenda? Given what I have just said, it might be foolish of me to generalize about this. I say this seriously, because I do not believe there is any "off-the-peg" solution; there can only be an aspiration, a determination to engage with something, a process. There can of course be defined goals, but to reach them requires a complex transformative process that cannot be known in advance.

I have one enduring image from the most intense period of our efforts to lead and facilitate development at the Tavistock. It is of myself and my two colleagues (one black, one white) who shared a post, funded by government to act as Race and Equity Training Development workers, huddled in my office week after week attempting to process our experience of the work. We often felt profoundly isolated, and even slightly crazy, struggling to find and hold on to confidence in our perception of the organizational turbulence we seemed to provoke, and to facilitate meaningful interventions against this background. Some of the more painful varieties of experience I recall from this period of work include:

» Finding close colleagues, who were ostensibly explicitly committed to the aims of improved race and equity relationships and provision, *behaving* in uncooperative, obstructive, and undermining ways.
» Experiencing other colleagues, whom I had assumed to be supporters of the project, as "silent", neutral, or uninterested.
» From time to time, experiencing myself/ourselves as the object of knotty, involved projective dynamics that sometimes took many months to make sense of, and then often inconclusively.

Were these unexpected dynamics rooted in covert resistance to the project of tackling issues of race in the organization, or merely continuations of more familiar rivalrous, territorial, competitive relationships, or both? It was impossible to know, mirroring perhaps a common uncertainty for ethnic minorities with respect to their experience of relationships with the majority community—is this racism, prejudice, or just an ordinary experience of competitive discomfort, exclusion in relation to the group? Consequently, I think we all experienced profound doubt at times about whether we were seeing the world straight, or not. Perhaps we were deluded and the institution perfectly sane? Previous experience of leading intensive group-training programmes on the dynamics of race was one source of support—we had been there before.

Here are two brief extracts from an earlier paper about these programmes of work (Cooper, 1997), undertaken with mixed-race groups of social work students, and facilitated by a mixed-race staff group:

> At the start of proceedings . . . I observed that it was noticeable that several of the black students in the group were not present. Later the same morning I was addressed directly by two white group members and told that in saying this I was "talking out of my arse".
>
> In the room are 30 students and four staff members. Seven of the students and one of the staff identify as black. I introduce this workshop and hand out lists of the four small groups, three for white students and one for black, in which we plan to work for much of the time. There are murmurings, questions. "Why have the groups been pre-selected?" I reply that we have used ordinary criteria, a reasonable distribution of the sexes and some attention to existing familiarities through other course groups. This does not satisfy the questioners. "All other groups on this course have been self-selecting" says one. This is about as far from the truth as is conceivable. . . . Perhaps it goes without saying that the students asking these questions are white. For the moment, no-one, or at least no white student, has caught on to the fact that given everyone had been told we would be working in same race groups, one group—the group of seven black students—is self-selecting. [Cooper, 1997, pp. 129–130]

My experience is that when someone comes out and *names* the fact of racial difference in an organizational context, even though these "differences" may be absolutely visible and evident to all, it often arouses intense anxiety for white members of the organization. For black or other visible ethnic minorities, hardly at all—they, after all, live with the awareness of the actual or potential implications of their visible difference every day. Simply announcing in an institution the intention to undertake a project or development in relation to "race" can, for this reason, arouse instantaneous resistance. I believe the anxiety often takes the form of a belief that black people will feel, or be, "exposed" as a result. But, in reality, what is "exposed" are profound anxieties for white people about what is involved in their own everyday "noticing" of difference. As one white member of the group described above later elaborated:

> Hesitatingly a white student begins to speak about what he says he has often thought but never voiced—that the black students in this course group tend to sit together. He continues, honestly if rather

> clumsily, to express his confusion about his awareness of black people's visible difference from white people. "I don't know how to deal with this" he says, "What do you say? Hello, black person?" [Cooper, 1997, p. 131]

The two students who accused me of "speaking out of my arse" have not processed their discomfort even to this point. They believe their attack on me will be supported and welcomed by their black colleagues, whom they take to have been "exposed" or affronted by my public naming of visible racial difference—they are quickly disillusioned by their black colleagues, who quietly express their sense that my remarks was perfectly appropriate in the context. In my experience, this "manoeuvre" in which a white person "allies" with a black colleague, to protect them against what they take to be the racist implications of "naming" difference by another white person, is a common variety of defence against the anxieties of beginning to explore race in group or organizational life. I understand it as a form of projection, in which deep fears about the impact of the racist unconscious (present, no doubt, in all dominant ethnic communities irrespective of "colour") are expelled into another member of the same community.

During the course of development work at the Tavistock and the BAP, I believe I and my colleagues were embroiled in more than one exchange that took the above form. In a draft of the original paper on which this chapter is based, I tried to describe in detail one such instance, in which I felt publicly humiliated and paralysed, as a colleague implied that some remarks I had made were racist and simultaneously "recruited" the one black person in the room to her view by saying she "could not imagine" what this black colleague must be feeling. But in the end I could reach no satisfactory understanding or agreement with the other party to the exchange about what had "happened", and so I was obliged not to include this account. This, again, is familiar. Organizational work on "race" mobilizes intensely persecutory states of mind and, not infrequently, leads towards "impasse". Replacing enactment with understanding may be very hard to achieve.

Theoretical resources are urgently needed if we are to find ways to help ourselves with such processes. I want to draw upon Fakhry Davids' work on the idea of the "internal racist" (Davids, 2003) to provide some help. The internal racist is an inner-world *relationship*, an object relationship, between an attacked and denigrated part of the self and a hostile and attacking one, but a relationship that takes a racialized shape or form. Typically, in our culture and epoch, the hostile figure may be "white" and the attacked and damaged figure "black", although this may be rapidly reversed in the manner so characteristic of inner-world functioning. When I spoke earlier of a dependent or emotionally needy part of the self being suppressed, controlled, or attacked from within, one can imagine such a relational configuration assuming a racialized form. This "internal organization" may often be quiescent, or it may be there in various forms of "hiding" behind or within other defensive structures in the personality that lend a hand in disguising its presence to the self and others. But it can be mobilized, brought to life in the self, and when this happens it causes anxiety. One solution to this anxiety is to project the entire organization into some outer-world receptacle. This is what I find so helpful about the notion—it is not "racist impulses" or "hatred" that is projected, but an entire relationship. This is what I believe may have taken place in the vignette I have just described.

Fakhry Davids makes it clear that in his view the internal racist is pretty much a universal phenomenon. We've all got one. I do not want to speak as though I believe I am exempt from this, so I will tell you a short and rather painful story from my own experience. I went to dinner with a friend and a couple of other people. My friend is of Middle-Eastern origin, dark-skinned but not black. It was summer, and the evening drew in as we were sitting round the table in subdued lighting. I suddenly noticed that my friend seemed to have dirty marks on her elbows. We had drunk a bit, or at least I had, and the conversation had turned to some light-hearted banter about the man who lived next door and whether my friend might find a way to get to know him better. There was a suggestion that she might find a pretext to visit him. Suddenly, thinking I was making a joke, I said, "Make sure you wash your elbows before you go". I don't really recall people's reaction at the time, but my friend phoned me the next day and very kindly said that she had found my remark really offensive. "Apart from anything else," she said "it was so racialized." Only then did it dawn on me that the marks on her elbows were pigmentation, dark local colouring of her skin.

There is much that could be unfolded out of this story, and in other published work Fakhry Davids has described with great clarity the way that skin colour can become projectively identified with psychic dirt—hostility and conflict—so that black children may believe their skin is "dirty". Anyone who has worked with black children in the care system will know that this is a common fantasy, sometimes leading to dangerous attempts to turn the skin "white". In a book chapter called "The Psychic Geography of Racism", Julian Lousada describes some sessions with a black patient who had been subjected in a public place to a sudden, unexpected verbally racist assault by a woman. A few days later, he meets her again. "Oh, I am so glad to see you, I wanted to apologise for my outburst I just went out of my mind", the woman says. The author comments:

> The racist thug would attack you in the street, he thought, fully conscious of his hatred even if not knowing why; while the woman's outburst of "hatred" was more like an ambush. To make matters worse he had come to understand that *both* he and this woman had been the subject of an ambush—she from within, and himself from without. At any moment and with only limited provocation the individual or group can self-evidently go out of its mind. [Cooper & Lousada, 2005, p. 89]

My own ashamed and rueful feeling on being phoned by my friend was also of having been ambushed from within. But then, we know this is how the unconscious works sometimes.

At the level of institutional life I want to propose that our internal racists are normally all pretty much quiescent or in hiding. Some of the features of organizational culture I have described—liberal tolerance, the belief in guardianship of special knowledge—are possibly excellent defensive hiding places for these structures. But open talk of the possibility of institutional racism, or of an initiative to achieve greater ethnic diversity, arouses these anxiety-laden structures. They surface more openly in organizational life, rather than creeping about in whispers in the corridors and informal spaces of the institution.

In the development work undertaken at the BAP, various working groups and seminars dedicated to the question of how to alter the ethnic balance of both the membership and the patient population had been in train for some time. Along the way, we found that several "stuck" situations cropped up. Pairs of white members became involved in rather intractable dynamics in which someone was accusing (or felt to be accusing) someone else of racism. Statements perceived by others as racist, but which may have gone unchallenged at the time, were made in groups and written up as part of the report of the work. What do we do with them? Suppress them, downplay them, publish them, challenge them *post facto*? The most tempting option in the face of all this is to retreat, close the lid on this can of worms, and comfort ourselves with the thought that "We tried".

Not giving up might be associated with the idea that there is another side to the toxic dynamics we encounter. Maybe we all have an internal racist, but maybe most of us have reparative, hopeful inner objects too. My mother died when she was 88. When she was about 84, I sat having a conversation with her one day, and out of nowhere she began to tell me that she had been a member of Anti-Apartheid for many years and, through them, had a regular correspondence with a black woman called Ruby who lived in Soweto. She showed me a photograph of her and some of the letters. I think this may have been the first time she had ever spoken to anyone in our family about this. It was a kind of secret life she led. She may have manifested a baffling lack of awareness about the naming of her chocolate-meringue puddings, but on the other hand she was engaged in a small, compassionate, secret, and, for her, rather subversive political project. When I reflect on my own disposition during my life to become involved in this area of work, I sometimes wonder whether this disposition is not an unconscious continuation of some unfinished project of my mother's.

Hiding places

In the work I was engaged in at the Tavistock, it often felt as though the central group carrying the leadership responsibility was about to implode, explode, or somehow fall apart. Certainly we often felt isolated, beleaguered, and very unloved. In a sense it did eventually dissolve after about five years, partly because of central NHS requirements that trusts should have a "single equalities scheme" rather than initiatives directed to particular inequalities. But not before a good deal had been achieved. I don't want to detail these achievements, or overestimate them, but the transformations that have been effected (and there are many that have not) do feel to be more or less irreversible. I was the most encouraged by a rather informal observation from a friend and colleague who visits the Tavistock only occasionally, with whom I was discussing this work. She said to me recently, "It just feels completely different when you go in there and walk around, from how it felt five years ago".

The institutions I have spoken about are not the only ones who have tackled similar projects in the area of race and equity. I just know less, or in some cases nothing of these. I don't want to be heard as representing their experiences, or indeed as misrepresenting and ignoring them. I have been trying to speak on the basis of what I think or hope I know something about. So, can psychotherapy, and psychotherapy institutions, change in the ways I have been discussing? Of course there is evidence that they can, and also evidence that some have not even started. In a way I have taken a long time to say something rather obvious—if you think there is a problem with your institution, it needs an *institutional* approach to tackle it. No amount of interesting, clever, insightful work based only on our essentially dyadic or triadic clinical–theoretical work will by itself achieve the task. And I have been saying that psychotherapists may not be very good at institutional life in certain important ways, for particular reasons associated with the very unusual nature of their work and of their core preoccupations.

If that is at all correct, they are both like the rest of humanity, as Farhad Dalal says, but also unlike them. That is what I believe to be the truth about all institutions and social formations. It is easier to grasp the "sameness", the universality; harder to really work with and face the differences, the particularity, the idiosyncratic, especially when it is alive, dynamic, and potentially destructive. But the choice is always the same: we can stay in hiding, or we can come out and engage, struggle. It's that simple and it's that difficult.

Note

1. Officially the Tavistock "Clinic" no longer exists. The clinic is one part of the Tavistock and Portman NHS Foundation Trust, a mental health trust within NHS mainstream provision, although its services and training provision continue to be distinctive.

CHAPTER SEVEN

Trauma, truth, and the court

Facts and fictions

What does a psychotherapist have to say that might conceivably be of interest to practitioners concerned with legal evidence and courtroom procedure? Respect for hard evidence is not, I suspect, something the public at large believes psychotherapists are much preoccupied with. Sometimes we even think this about ourselves. There is an "in" joke about one of the founders of modern psychoanalysis. Her patient is late for a session, and she is displeased. "You are ten minutes late", she says to the patient when he eventually fetches up, "You have missed the first two interpretations."

If we are sometimes accused of arriving at interpretations on the basis of insufficient evidence, then occasionally the classic texts do rather support this view. Freud's famous and lengthy case study of the "Wolf Man" culminates in an evidential *tour de force*. From the Wolf Man's clinical material, and from his celebrated childhood dream—of waking at night and seeing his bedroom window open of its own accord to reveal six or seven white wolves sitting very still—Freud reconstructs the traumatic moment of origin of his patient's afflictions with astonishing precision; namely that at the age of one and a half, on a summer's afternoon—probably at about five o'clock—he woke in his cot and witnessed his parents having sexual intercourse three times. Freud even deduces the position in which they coupled—the detail is relevant to the reconstruction—but rather coyly protects the reader from the full impact of this knowledge by sometimes rendering it in Latin—"*a tergo, more ferarum*" (Freud, 1918b).

The methodology of psychoanalysis as represented in these case studies has often been likened to detective work—or is it detective fiction? This ambiguity lies at the root of the numerous works of detective fiction that have been inspired by psychoanalysis. The *Interpretation of Murder*, a fictional reworking of Freud's case study of Dora (1905e), authored by an American Professor of Law (Rubenfeld, 2007), is one example. More seriously, Wilfred Bion, who was deeply concerned to get to the bottom of the question of what we can really know, said in a short paper entitled "Evidence",

> I sometimes think that a feeling is one of the few things which analysts have the luxury of being able to regard as a fact. If patients [and I think he might have added, therapists themselves] are feeling angry, or frightened, or sexual, or whatever it is, at least we can suppose that this is a fact; but when they embark on theories or hearsay we cannot distinguish fact from fiction. [Bion, 1994, p. 317]

Truth—historical and psychic

Contemporary clinical theory and practice now tends to occupy a position somewhere between the assumptions driving Freud's effort at total reconstruction of "historical truth", and Bion's pure phenomenology of the "affective moment". In truth, Freud himself led us towards this stance. His so-called abandonment of the "seduction theory" of the aetiology of the cases of female hysteria that were so important to his early work—broadly that an actual experience of sexual abuse or trauma lay at the root of the problem—in favour of an explanation in terms of the patient's guilty and hence repressed *fantasy* of some seduction, ushers in the notion of "psychic reality" or "psychic truth". On this view, our conscious and unconscious thoughts, beliefs, memories, and representations of our experience are always in some measure a mixture of "fact" and "fantasy". As Freud says,

> Up to the present we have not succeeded in pointing to any difference in the consequences, whether phantasy or reality has had the greater share in these events of childhood. [Freud, 1916–17, p. 370]

Thus psychoanalysis sets out with the assumption that the patient's neurotic symptoms are grounded at least in psychic reality and that in this sense, "the patient must surely be right in some way" (Freud, 1917e, p. 246). "In some way . . ." Here, I think the world of the consulting room and the world of the courtroom both meet and go their separate ways. In various respects, it is the simultaneous differentiation of, and interplay between, "historical truth" and "psychic truth" that is the central theme of this chapter.

Early in his thinking, Freud thought that some form of "trauma" lay at the root of most if not all neurotic difficulties. Today, while actual trauma, including childhood sexual trauma, has certainly been reinstated as hugely significant in our understanding of the aetiology of many kinds of mental health difficulties, we also know that traumatic experiences typically have particular and distinctive consequences for the growth and development of the mind. Equally, not every patient coming into therapy has experienced trauma, unless one widens the definition of that term in an unhelpful manner. As one of my clinical supervisors during my training put it to me, "Some people suffer from trauma, some from conflict, and some from misconceptions". Of course, this is just a useful little rule of thumb, and many patients are afflicted by all three, and more.

Trauma, truth, and memory: some clinical vignettes

Before I turn to consider some particular implications of traumatized mind states for forensic and courtroom evidential procedure, I want to give a flavour from clinical practice of how relationships between trauma, historical truth, and psychic truth can manifest themselves.

A patient who had been physically abused as a child came to a session one day and recounted a memory of how his father had beaten him severely at the age of about 4 years because he had lost control of his bladder and bowels on a visit to some relatives. As is often the case when patients recount such experiences, I had a powerful sense not so much that he was remembering these events for the first time, but that they were being recollected and recounted with a new kind of emotional focus or steadiness afforded perhaps by the safety of the therapeutic relationship. The following day, he came to his session and described how he had thought about this memory overnight, and that it now seemed to him that probably events had been the other way round in certain respects. He now thought that his father had become angry with him, perhaps because he had been pestering to go home, and had beaten him, as a result of which he had lost control of his bowels and bladder.

In his everyday adult life, this man was often prey to the kind of confusion about time, event sequences, causality, and attributions of responsibility for events that characterize the uncertainty of perspective in his childhood memory of traumatic events. He once described how he had arrived for an appointment with an academic supervisor and, finding the room empty, had panicked and jumped to the conclusion that the appointment had been the previous day, that his supervisor must be furious, and that his career was in jeopardy as a result. He went to his office and began writing a letter of apology, when the supervisor phoned to enquire where he was. As these experiences unfolded in the therapy, I was able to make more sense of my first meeting with him. He had an appointment for a consultation at 4.00 pm. At 3.15 my doorbell rang, and I found him on the doorstep apologizing profusely for being a quarter of an hour late.

As a therapist I was convinced I was hearing about "real events" in the examples just given: that the childhood beating had occurred in pretty much the circumstances described, just as the visit to the supervisor's office had. I was also persuaded that the patient's revised account of his childhood experience was probably the more accurate; and that his capacity to "recover", not memory itself, but a more veridical account of who had done what to whom in what order, with all the attendant implications about agency and responsibility that these details imply, was important in his recovery process in therapy. A core of "historical truth" seems to be preserved intact. But the systematic distortions or displacements of sequence, causality, and so on in both the remembered account and in contemporary functioning have an almost delusional quality. Events are transcribed so that the man himself is always in the wrong and is profoundly anxious that he is about to be punished.

However, this constellation of mind states could take a different turn. On one occasion, I had to alter the usually stable arrangements of the therapy at rather short notice. He came to the session in a fury, absolutely convinced that this was a malign and manipulative plot to in some way test his commitment to the therapy. His conviction dissipated gradually, but for a time it had the fixed certainty of a delusion. I shall return to the judicial significance of such states of mind later in the chapter.

Another brief clinical example emphasizes a slightly different dimension of traumatic experience. A young woman whose studies sometimes involve working with heavy machinery described an experience of intrusive fantasies of placing her hand in one of the machines so that it would be mangled. Towards the end of the two-day period in which she was working in this particular environment, she then "accidentally" cut her hand very badly with a sharp implement, but nevertheless insisted on driving herself to hospital to get treatment. As she recounted these events in therapy, the woman linked them to facts and memories of which I had previously heard nothing. When she was about 10 years old, her father had been seriously ill and this had resulted in him losing several of the fingers of one hand.

For me, there was again a sense not of "recovered memory" in the ordinary sense of the term, but of a "recovering emotional memory": a process in which the impact of these childhood events—fear that her father was dying, anxieties about whether she had in some way contributed to his illness and damage—could now find a place in her adult mind where they could be *thought about*. Unable to assimilate the intensity of these anxieties at the time, she could not properly symbolize or narrate this whole area of experience; nevertheless, the memory remains alive and active, and is first of all *enacted* until, in the presence of another mind able to tolerate and in some measure take in and process the emotional meaning of the experience with her, it can be assimilated as a part of the adult personality. This, I hope, gives a picture of how therapists think about trauma, memory, emotion, enactment, and our part in trying to help people afflicted by such experiences.

From even this brief exploration, there would seem to be potentially wide-ranging implications for forensic and courtroom procedure, and for concepts of "evidence". I shall attempt to draw out just some of these that I hope will be of value in the proceedings of the conference.

The traumatized witness

I ask myself, "What kind of witness or defendant would someone afflicted by these sorts of mind states make in court?" Or at least, since the states of mind described above are often partially or wholly "encapsulated" within otherwise cognitively well-functioning people, what kind of witness would they make in relation to events that resonated with or evoked anxieties of a parallel kind? The examples of trauma I have offered are not especially severe. In both instances, however, we see something of the complex interplay between what are called, in the jargon, explicit and implicit, and declarative and non-declarative, memory. In more severe trauma, this may underlie what we ordinarily think of as traumatic amnesia. As one set of commentators have summarized it:

> Trauma can differentially affect explicit and implicit memory. The nonverbal (nondeclarative) aspects of the experience, such as the fear response, may be encoded as implicit memory, while the verbal aspects (i.e. the comments of the perpetrator, the victim's inner dialog during the experience, the narrative of the experience) may not be encoded. According to recent neuropsychological findings, the fact that the declarative or narrative aspects of the traumatic experience *may* not be encoded as explicit memory is due to disruption of the functions of the hippocampus in the brain. This hippocampus dysfunction, in turn, is linked to the high level of stress neurohormones produced during serious traumas. At the same time, the perceptual, physiological, emotional, and motor aspects of the traumatic experience, and particularly the fear response, are recorded in other neural maps involving the amygdala (which, unlike the hippocampus, is not affected by the stress neurohormones). Therefore, the traumatic experience cannot be retrieved in any narrative form during verbal interchanges concerning the patient's memories. While the body memory of the trauma persists in the form of phobias and psychosomatic disturbances, the traumatic experience may never become part of autobiographical memory. [Liotti, Mollon, & Miti, 2007, p. 204]

As a result of trauma a patient, defendant, or witness may have no narrative recall of key events that a layperson might think likely to be especially memorable. Equally, as we have seen, they may have such recall but offer significantly different versions of it at different times; or they may render a (probably) false account of such events with absolute conviction. Was the first patient I described lying, or dissembling, on either occasion he recounted his childhood experience? I don't think so. As Freud said, "The patient must surely be right in some way." Would someone afflicted by such experiential uncertainty about events make a credible witness in court? Probably not. Might they nevertheless deserve a hearing as part of proceedings? Very possibly.

IICSA and the contemporary relevance of "therapeutic justice"

The arguments of this chapter are relevant to the experiences of everyone involved in what is possibly the most radical and ambitious judicial–therapeutic project ever launched in the United Kingdom—the Independent Inquiry into Child Sexual Abuse (IICSA). In particular, the strand of this inquiry known as the Truth Project, in which individuals have the opportunity to narrate their experiences of historic institutional sexual abuse to trained staff acting in a non-judicial role, facilitates communications in which the boundary between psychological, historical, and evidential registers of "truth" are acceptably blurred and are not a "problem" in terms of their status as evidence. Experiential truth is privileged over any other variety.

For the facilitators and others who receive those coming forward and listen to their accounts, the experience can be emotionally and personally testing. Many of the stories involve harrowing details of extreme cruelty, violence, and physical and psychological intrusion and exploitation by adults of the child, now an adult him/herself, sitting before them. Intense feelings of fear, terror, abandonment, psychological annihilation, disgust, and incomprehension are evoked in the here-and-now of the Truth session. These sessions are not therapy, although they may result in some degree of psychological relief for survivors and victims; importantly, they seem to entail a sense of being "heard" by an institution that is formally mandated by the state. Facilitators often report that participants leave sessions visibly "lighter" and physically less burdened than when they arrived. My belief is that it is the capacity of facilitators to genuinely take in the depth and intensity of emotional experience being communicated that accounts not just for this visible impact, but also for the sense that finally someone has been able to "bear witness".

Truth sessions are audio-recorded, and the assistant facilitator takes contemporaneous notes. The records of sessions will become data in the wide-ranging research programme connected to the inquiry. Summary narratives of early Truth sessions are published on the IICSA website (https://www.iicsa.org.uk), although they have been strikingly leached of their powerful and immediate emotional content. Nevertheless this entire project represents a remarkably different way of "doing justice to" a pervasive, socially toxic, and profoundly individually damaging aspect of our social and institutional life, which has consequences for huge numbers of ordinary citizens. Viewed like this, the project constitutes a further step in the gradual, uncertain process of our society becoming capable of facing and tolerating the "dangerous knowledge" of terrible things that are happening for people all around us—"just down the street", as I put it at one point in this book (see chapter 12); as with the other landmark processes in the history of child protection in this country discussed in chapter 8, a state apparatus is essential to enable "an apparatus for thinking" and action at a social and political level. Equally the principles and practices embodied in the work of the Truth Project constitute an example of social policy operating as a "social container" for emotionally charged individual and social experience, with the prospect that this depth engagement with lived experience may ultimately deliver policy responses better attuned to—because shaped by—these experiences, rather than the familiar application of "instrumental reason" to "social problems" so characteristic of traditional policymaking. These matters are more fully explored in chapter 10.

The traumatized offender

Do those who have suffered trauma at the hands of others receive understanding and a fair deal in our criminal courts? I offer two kinds of answer to this rather large question.

As clinicians, much of the trauma that we hear about from adult patients, or in relation to which we intervene in the lives of children and young people, is best thought of as "cumulative trauma" (Khan, 1986). Some of the best research evidence we now have for the aetiology of serious adult mental health disorders concerns the damaging impact on the development of the minds of infants of frightening and/or frightened care-giving, and the subsequent consequences of this. Infants and young children who have received such care are prone to develop what we call "disorganized attachment patterns", and in turn these predict patterns of controlling and aggressive behaviour in later childhood and in adulthood. Adults diagnosed with Borderline Personality Disorder (BPD) often have this kind of history. Not everyone with such a history becomes violent or an offender of any kind—far from it. But, our prisons are full of people—mainly men, of course—with very serious mental health problems of this kind. For most of them, if we care to look, there is a story of serious childhood developmental difficulties involving what we could think of as cumulative trauma. Often I suspect this is obscured by the other histories they have—of drug dependency, alcoholism, gang membership, and so on. But all these people have passed through our courts. I have little doubt that most of them are guilty of the crimes for which they have been convicted. A fair proportion of them are, for want of a more judicious way of expressing it, extremely unpleasant people. But then I think of the definition of mental illness that Donald Winnicott attributes to his psychoanalyst friend John Rickman: "Mental illness consists in not being able to find anyone who can stand you" (Winnicott, 1965, p. 218).

Earlier, I tried to articulate something about the connection between traumatization, subsequent difficulties in being able to symbolize, narrate, or in ordinary language "reflect on and think about" the experiences involved, the inevitability of confused and confusing enactments of the trauma in the subject's life, and the role of the therapist in providing a thinking mind that can begin to "process" traumatic experience and allow it to be better integrated.

Recent research into the nature and treatment of BPD refines this view somewhat. Cumulative trauma in childhood leads to the child internalizing the frightening or hostile mind states of the caretaker; it also engenders a failure of development of "self-reflective function", or capacity for "mentalization"—broadly a capacity to distinguish self and other and to think clearly about who is doing what to whom for what reason in interpersonal relationships. Burdened with intolerable emotional mind states, such people seek out others to, as it were, "carry" some of this emotional burden. Thus:

> Acts of violence may occur if an attempt at externalisation fails. If the other refuses to be cowed or humiliated into becoming a vehicle for intolerable self-states, the individual with severe personality disorder frequently turns to interpersonal destruction. [Bateman & Fonagy, 2006, p. 27]

The same authors describe what they call "psychic equivalence", a state of mind typical of borderline functioning, especially when the defensive structures that protect the individual are threatened.

> The first formulation to emerge in one's mind is the only possible formulation; it cannot be questioned; no information can be provided that would shift or dislodge that attitude. The affective tone induced by psychic equivalence is commonly characterized by paranoid hostility. [Bateman & Fonagy, 2006, p. 21]

This was more or less the state of mind the man described above manifested on the occasion when I altered his session time. When traumatic enactments have led to actual criminal acts, we may think that the person's subsequent denials of responsibility or his or her systematic distortions of the apparent reality of who was responsible for what took place are conscious and cunning efforts to deflect blame and avoid judicial consequences. Frequently, the situation may be quite different. The subject *really does believe* that the victim in effect perpetrated the crime through provocation, for example. The delusional belief protects him or her from experiencing states of mind that are felt to be even more catastrophic.

Writing in a publication about interdisciplinary work in the family justice system, Carola Thorpe extends these points:

> The perpetrator's acts often disgust us, but we have learnt to understand that such acts are born of attempts by the perpetrator to manage his/her own troubled interior life. These attempts are usually futile psychologically in that they circumvent the core distress that is too painful to admit into consciousness. And because the hoped for relief is not achieved, except perhaps briefly, it has to be repeated. [Thorpe, 2007, p. xiv]

Of course, other criminological perspectives might see it very differently, but my point in this part of the chapter is that a large part of the criminal justice system is arguably taken up with processing the consequences—the truth, if you like—of trauma.

Children and the family court

Trauma does, I believe, receive a different kind of hearing in the family courts than in the criminal courts. This is partly because the task is different, and children of all ages are the object of concern. Accordingly, court procedures and processes are different and follow a more inquisitorial model. Lord Justice Wall has summarized this:

> The family court has the advantage, denied to criminal lawyers, that the rules of evidence are relaxed. Whilst the court exercises a fierce control over who is shown the court papers, and which experts are called to give evidence, hearsay evidence is admitted . . . judges are entitled to garner evidence from all sources they think will assist. The reasons for the different approaches are obvious. Criminal courts are concerned with the right of the state to punish individuals if an offence has been committed. It follows that the offence must be strictly proved. Family courts are concerned with child protection. [Wall, 2007, pp. 17–18]

Here is an extract from a clinical account by a child psychotherapist of an assessment she did for the family court and her commentary on this material:

> Two little girls, aged 2 and 4, come to the consulting room and immediately notice that there is no handle on the door to the room. (Some repair work was being undertaken in the clinic.) They are preoccupied with this and it reflects, quite by chance, something from their own experience. They had, in reality, been kept locked in a room by their mother who had removed the door handle on the inside so that they could not get out. This meant that they were stuck

> with each other and their own excrement that was smeared on the walls. . . . What the older child said was that they had been alone in an empty room and they couldn't get out, not even to go to the toilet. She said that the two of them played with the pet hamster, throwing it around and banging it against the walls until it died. The older child said it was the younger one who had killed it; the younger child did not speak.
>
> According to the "facts" from the external world, what had actually happened was that the children had been left in a room unable to get out and that faeces had been smeared on the walls. However, the hamster had died in very different circumstances from those communicated by the older child in the consulting room. The adults had been in the front room and the two children were scooting around in a plastic sit-in car, one inside and the other pushing. The hamster was not in its cage and it got run over. Why should the children tell such a different story?
>
> When I reflected on the difference between the two stories of the hamster's death, one the "truth" of *external reality* and the other the "lie" the children had told, I thought about it in terms of the children's actual experience: whilst they may have had adults present in the room with them when the hamster actually died, effectively they were alone and that is what was said. Perhaps the truth is worse than the "lie"—the adults present were unable to take protective action to prevent a hamster dying. In their *internal reality* the children were alone in the room with the hamster when it died.
>
> In this case the child psychotherapist could give the court a vivid picture of neglect and harm suffered by the children, despite arguments in defence of the mother aiming to minimise her responsibility and blame the children for being naughty and smearing the walls. [Tydeman, 2007, pp. 36–37]

Therapeutic work can corroborate other "findings of fact" and, in turn, be corroborated by these, but it can also throw up material that seems puzzling and anomalous and that might, under other circumstances, cast doubt on the reliability of such testimony. In this case the therapist makes *emotional* sense of the aspects of the children's story that don't "fit the facts" and found she could deploy this as evidence

Reflecting more generally, Beverley Tydeman says:

> What we discover about the child's inner world during our assessment sessions usually illuminates what is already known from more external sources that are present as "facts" in the bundle. These "facts" are brought to light through the child's communication with the therapist in the consulting room. As an expert witness this is then brought to life by the descriptions that the child psychotherapist

> gives to the court. . . . The court wants to know that our perceptions are based on clinical "facts" and are not distorted by our own internal prejudices, weaknesses, blind spots or preferences. [Tydeman, 2007, p. 36]

English family court practice is slowly taking shape as genuinely interdisciplinary and honed to the particular circumstances of the work it does. Lord Justice Wall again:

> . . . I have developed a considerable faith in what I can best describe as interdisciplinary good practice, and that in my court I expected the work of the medical and psychiatric expert to be examined rigorously. . . . That process, conducted with courtesy, and combined with an equally rigorous forensic examination of the facts usually enabled me to reach a conclusion which I could live with . . . [Wall, 2007, p. 13]

Concluding thoughts

Does this mean that the tension between forensic or historical truth and evidence on the one hand, and psychic truth on the other, has been somehow resolved in these forums? Not entirely, I suspect, since I further suspect that they do reflect irreducibly different ways of understanding and conceptualizing psychological and social realities. One moment in Beverly Tydeman's discourse betrays the continuing tension: she refers to the child's version of the death of the hamster as a "lie" (albeit with speech marks), yet she is at pains to emphasize that this story represents the child's psychic truth.

So much of what happens in court seems to depend on the reliability of testimony, and memory. Yet we know from research, and experience, that everyday normal "autobiographical memory" is hopelessly "unreliable" with respect to ordinary historical truth (Mollon, 2002). Paradoxically, from a psychological standpoint, this is an aspect of mental health, as opposed to disturbance. Traumatic memory is often seemingly "fixed" and repetitive, impervious to the influence of "suggestion and incorporation of new information from various sources" (Liotti, Mollon, & Miti, 2007, p 204), although this does not mean it is any more veridical with respect to the "facts" of what happened.

"Evidence" seems to be a complex, uncertain, ambiguous, and shifting concept, and an equally complex and uncertain phenomenon in its own right. Trauma makes this more so. And yet, as I hope to have shown, trauma is frequently at the very heart of the matters that our criminal and family justice systems deal in day by day.

PART III

POLITICS, POLICY, AND CULTURE

CHAPTER EIGHT

A short psycho-social history of British child abuse and protection

Introduction

If we step back and try to understand, as a total situation, the phenomenon of child maltreatment and child protection work in England in the twenty-first century, then what do we see? Self-evidently, we are confronted with a cultural and political phenomenon and not just a professional, legal, familial, or social-scientific one. In this sense, child abuse and protection are not unique. Other practices addressed to difficult human predicaments, and which were once largely the preserve of specialized professional, legal, and scientific systems, have escaped the boundaries of these same systems and become a focus of intense public, political, and cultural debate and anxiety. Autism and its putative link to the MMR vaccine is one instance. Human embryo research and the ethics of human tissue preservation are another. In all such cases where professional and scientific practices are suddenly propelled into the turbulence of the public sphere, the consequences for practitioners, for the ethics of professional conduct, and for the research methodology itself are surely acute and often irreversible. Following a public crisis of these kinds in the domain of the practice concerned, things are never the same again. Such events are rather like a trauma to a hitherto stable professional system.

Eileen Munro's series of reports (Munro, 2010, 2011a, 2011b) into the British child protection system, and the reforms that she proposed, relied heavily on a systemic analysis of both the problems and solutions. Her arguments are detailed, rigorous, well evidenced, and persuasive and, at the time of writing, have undoubtedly led to an improved climate for child protection work in Britain. In the context of the historical perspective taken in this chapter, her explanation of the repetitive public crises afflicting the system is interesting:

> When society was outraged by the death of Maria Colwell and the series of high profile cases through the 1970s and 1980s, professionals responded by gradually lowering the threshold for intervention to minimise the chances of missing another child in such extreme danger. This necessarily led to more families with low actual levels of abuse being caught up in the net. The cases of Cleveland and Orkney were unsurprising consequences: on these occasions, professionals were criticised for intervening inappropriately and removing large numbers of children from their homes unnecessarily. [Munro, 2010, p. 23]

This is one instance among many she offers of the operation of the law of unintended consequences in systems, and here she deploys it to account for the episodic recurrence of child protection crises in the public sphere.

My own perspective in this chapter is different, but not in contradiction with Munro's. Its main themes concern processes, over extended periods of time, of apparent social, professional, and intellectual resolution of key conflicts and debates about the nature and existence of some categories of child maltreatment, as well as processes of irresolution and repetition in relation to some other categories of child abuse. In some instances, the central controversy and the attendant public anxiety and entanglement with this is, as it were, laid to rest. In others, it keeps coming back to life. I characterize these processes in terms of a philosophical public dialogue between the specialized professional systems of child protection and the wider public sphere. I then enquire into some explanations for continued contestation and public anxiety around some categories of abuse and suggest that these have much to do with issues about the handling of death and mourning in the contemporary public and private spheres.

In the few years since the publication of Munro's reports, there has not been a recurrence of the kind of moral panic that attended the deaths of Victoria Climbié or Peter Connelly, despite fresh disturbing disclosures of the systematic abuse of vulnerable girls and of institutional collusion with these practices. There is evidence, for example, in the establishment of the government's Independent Inquiry into Child Sexual Abuse (https://www.iicsa.org.uk/), of development in our social capacity for thoughtful rather than reactive responses to revelations of hitherto unsuspected forms of abuse in our society. So, has there been a decisive shift in public and political mood, a greater acceptance that "mistakes will sometimes happen" and that, as Munro puts it, "prediction and prevention of child maltreatment is necessarily a fallible process" (2011a, p. 96), thus lowering the temperature in the public sphere sufficiently to avoid the need for further eruptions of public anxiety or moral panics, as they are often labelled?

Despite the parallels with episodes of public turbulence and scrutiny of specialized professional practices in other domains, I believe that this wider cultural history of English child maltreatment and protection and its consequences for everyday practice is distinctive and probably unique. I want to suggest that child protection controversies constitute a "limit case" of the processes I have alluded to above and that careful analysis of the complex dynamics involved may yield findings of much wider social significance.

The two tasks of the child protection system

What is a system of child protection for? What is a system for the protection of any group of vulnerable people for? I want to propose that it has at least two primary tasks, but that the tension between these can be a source of acute difficulties, and that in the English child protection system this tension lies at the heart of a real crisis. The crisis takes the form of a paradox or contradiction—in fact, a number of paradoxes. On many indices, including international comparisons, the system does quite well at protecting children from extreme and life-threatening abuse and violence. Research by Colin Pritchard and Richard Williams (2010) suggests that child abuse-related deaths in the UK have been declining steadily for the last 30 years and at a significantly higher rate of decline than all causes of child death. But the experience of those working in the system is different: from the perspective of front-line workers, and their managers, it is teetering on the brink of collapse, hanging on by its fingertips. And this experience has been getting steadily worse. Why is this?

In the week when the "Baby P" crisis was at its height in 2010, I wrote an article in a national newspaper and found myself engaged in a number of media appearances as a result. The most intelligent conversation I felt I had all week was with a London cab driver as I was on my way to a radio interview. I was apprehensive about his reaction when I told him what I was about to do—London cabbies not being especially well known for their liberal views. But he said, "I can't read about that case in the papers—it's too distressing. . . . I couldn't do that job, I wouldn't be able to sleep at night." He laughed a little nervously and looked at me in the mirror and said, "I suppose I wouldn't have been a very good social worker." But he had his finger on something important. One thing social workers and others in the child protection system do at a societal level is help people sleep at night—not because we are defending the realm against communists, terrorists, or insurgents, but because we are protecting people from the emotional impact of knowing about the torture and murder of babies that may be happening just down the street from where each of us lives.

Thus, my hypothesis is that the covert or unconscious primary task of the child protection system is to manage, on behalf of the rest of adult society, our deep ambivalence about children, about parenting, and about the propensity in all of us to feel like doing violence towards our own children—in other words, the ubiquity of hatred within the ordinary, everyday job of parenting. This is a largely unacknowledged reality in our society, and a difficult one to "evidence". Here I offer just one or two morsels, starting with a few lines from the novelist Rachel Cusk's (2002) uncomfortably honest book about her experience of motherhood:

> Looking after children is a low-status occupation. It is isolating, frequently boring, relentlessly demanding and exhausting. It erodes your self-esteem and your membership of the adult world. The more it is separated from the rest of life, the harder it gets. . . . As a mother you learn what it is to be both martyr and devil. In motherhood I have experienced myself as both more virtuous and more terrible, and more implicated too in the world's virtue and terror, than I would from the anonymity of childlessness have thought possible. [Cusk, 2002, pp. 7–8]

However, for a significant proportion of the population, official or media recognition of child maltreatment will not be functioning as a vehicle to assuage conscious or unconscious *anxieties* or fears ("It's ok, the actual abusers are over there and being dealt with by those social workers"), but as a representation of real experiences of abuse, known to them, but not disclosed or investigated, and hence beneath the surface of public awareness. How come?

> Child maltreatment remains a major public-health and social-welfare problem in high-income countries. Every year, about 4–16% of children are physically abused and one in ten is neglected or psychologically abused. During childhood, between 5% and 10% of girls and up to 5% of boys are exposed to penetrative sexual abuse, and up to three times this number are exposed to any type of sexual abuse. However, official rates for substantiated child maltreatment indicate less than a tenth of this burden. [Gilbert et al., 2008, p. 68]

So, up to ten times the amount of child abuse ever reported or investigated in Britain is lurking somewhere just beneath public, judicial, community, or professional awareness. What might be the contribution of the population of abusing adults, and young people, as well as unidentified victims of abuse, to eruptions of public outrage and anxiety when a child abuse case hits the headlines? In her psychoanalytic study of the Paulsgrove Estate anti-paedophile vigilante movement, Jessica Evans (2003) reveals that a high proportion of the women who whipped up the campaign against a fantasized "list" of locally resident paedophiles were themselves well known to children's services because of child care concerns:

> The women made definite secondary gains from putting themselves in the position of the persecuted, once they had projected all the destructiveness onto the paedophile other. Strengthened by the group, individuals achieved a position of moral rectitude that left them feeling omnipotent, and in control. [Evans, 2003, p. 177]

If we extend the principles of this analysis, then a further unacknowledged primary task of the child protection system is not just to be a container for universal anxieties and ambivalence of the kind that Rachel Cusk gives voice to, but as a site for the collective projection of denial of anxiety about actual abuse that goes unreported or uninvestigated. Alongside our more "ordinary" anxieties about hostility and aggression towards our own vulnerable and dependent children, so much actual child maltreatment, current and historical, remains a matter of secrecy, locked up within the closed family or the institutional systems that form around abusers and abused. When the professional system "fails" to contain or manage the difficult task of exposing and responding to maltreatment, and our wider society becomes temporarily embroiled in these matters, intense anxieties about the exposure of long-suppressed secret and dangerous knowledge of abuse are mobilized.

Truth, knowledge, and fantasy: a social dialogue

(a) The Cleveland crisis

I suggest that each time society is confronted anew with awareness of something like the actual prevalence of abuse in its midst, the impact of this new knowledge is traumatic in some meaningful sense of that rather abused word. Of course, the truly traumatic events—such as the widespread intra-familial sexual abuse of children—have already occurred; however, our collective capacity to tolerate *knowing* about this may not be securely established, so much so that there may not even be a language, an available conceptual apparatus or discourse, with which individuals or society can think about such matters. A kind of social repression barrier is operating.

I suggested earlier that the consequences of repeated explosions of public and political concern about single cases of child abuse or death have been negative for the capacity of the professional system to function. But there is another side to the story. In Figure 8.1, I represent what I see as certain very turbulent, but positive processes in which the specialized system of child protection was pressed into a complex philosophical dialogue with the remainder of society. The Cleveland crisis of 1987 is the first example. With Cleveland there really was a world before and a world after. In the course of a few turbulent months as the extraordinary events in Cleveland unfolded, our world changed, and changed, I believe, decisively for the better. The fact of widespread intra-familial sexual abuse in our society became established and broadly accepted. But not without a tremendous struggle: I think it is easy to forget how ill equipped we were in 1987 as a society and as individuals to cope with the emergence into social awareness of this most disturbing of social facts. In retrospect, it can seem as though a capacity to tolerate painful and unwelcome truths won out in a contest with the impulse to deny them and to label the truth-seekers mad. While this is accurate, and this was a crisis in which an opportunity for civilized progress was seized, I also believe we forget that at the time most of us were truly uncertain about the status of the disclosures and revelations that were emerging. Sexual abuse as a widespread social reality was breaking through a social repression barrier.

However, I believe that Cleveland became a social "crisis" not just because new and disturbing facts were emerging into the daylight, but

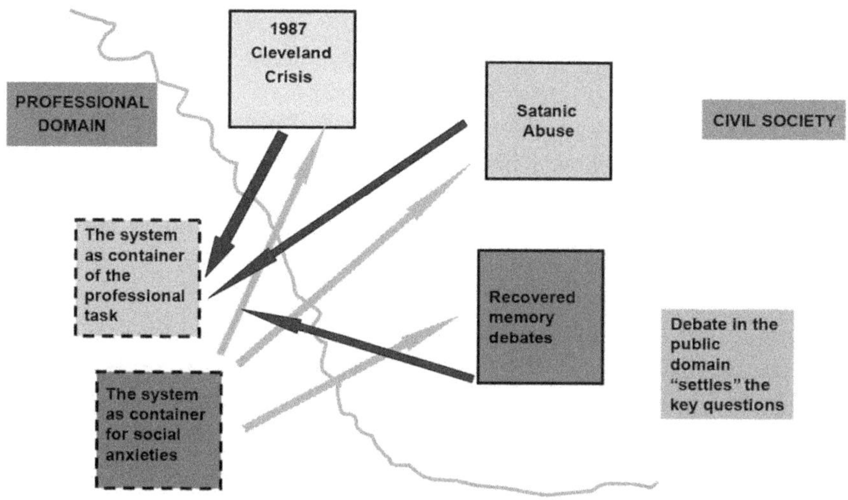

FIGURE 8.1. The two systems and the public sphere as a process of epistemological testing: What is true? What kinds of abuse exist or not?

also because these "facts" sometimes transpire to be *inherently* uncertain in their nature, independently of any social, political, ideological, or organizational pressure brought to bear by interested parties in the context of their emergence. In certain circumstances in sexual abuse, no one, not even the victim, may be sure "what happened". This fact—the fact of inherent possible indeterminacy or undecidability with respect to historical truths about abuse—seems to me to be an important but under-recognized component in the construction of the crisis. We like, or even need, to have a sense of certainty about such profound matters—true, false, it happened, it didn't happen. It may be true, as Freud claimed, that the incest taboo is the foundation stone of civilization, securing the boundary between reality-based and fantasy-based social and psychological functioning, but it then follows that where this boundary has been violated, something fundamental about our grip on the epistemological foundations of civilization will be compromised. This is a pretty frightening discovery. The predicament is alluded to in the report of the public inquiry into the Cleveland affair:

> The concept of helping the child to tell [of sexual abuse] is recognised to have its uses in certain circumstances. When embarking on it for diagnostic purposes, it is important to remember at least three possible situations:

> 1. The abuse has occurred and the child is speaking of it.
> 2. The abuse has occurred and the child is unable to speak of it or is denying it.
> 3. The abuse has not occurred, and the child cannot speak of it.
>
> It is clearly a difficult matter of judgement to know whether the child is not telling because of some sort of pressure, such as fear of the consequences, or because there is nothing to tell. At the end of a session, the professionals may not know which of those two situations is the true position. [HMSO, 1988, pp. 206–207]

However, after a period of testing in the public domain, the courts, and the inquiry process itself, something like a "true" overall position was settled upon. A large majority of cases of suspected sexual abuse in Cleveland were deemed to have been based in some reality. The Butler-Sloss inquiry effectively "settled" the contest about whether intra-familial sexual abuse was a "fantasy" or a "reality", and there has been no subsequent publicly endorsed effort to overturn this "settlement".

(b) Satanic abuse

The second episode concerns what became known as "Satanic abuse". This, as some may recall, was one dimension of the Orkneys crisis, but there were other sites of alleged exposure of Satanic abuse—especially in Rochdale and Nottingham. If the fact, the existence or otherwise, of child sexual abuse was temporarily and fiercely contested during the Cleveland affair, then the Satanic abuse disclosures led to even more controversial contestations. Broadly, and I suspect correctly, the weight of official evidence and opinion eventually settled on a judgement that the most extreme features of allegations of Satanic abuse were a kind of hysteria or group fantasy, but, along the way, some careful distinctions were established. The evidence for ritual abuse, and systems of organized child abuse, became better accepted and understood, but the more lurid allegations associated with Satanic abuse—sacrificial baby murder, cannibalism, drinking the blood of murdered children—were rejected. In thorough international studies, not a single shred of forensic evidence was discovered to support these claims. There are some respectable child mental health professionals who would dispute this outcome even today. Who is actually right, if there is an absolute right and wrong in this very murky area, is a matter of great importance. But in this chapter I am more interested in describing the rather unusual processes via which the questions involved are "tested".

To give us a flavour of where the controversy came to rest, here is one of the conclusions of Jean La Fontaine's research study, commissioned by government to try to investigate the allegations and settle the debate:

> 3. Rites that allegedly include the torture and sexual abuse of children and adults, forced abortion and human sacrifice, cannibalism and bestiality may be labelled satanic or Satanist. *Their defining characteristic is that the sexual and physical abuse of children is part of rites directed to a magical or religious objective. There is no evidence that these have taken place in any of the 84 cases studied.* [La Fontaine, 1994, p. 30; emphasis in original]

So, we are in familiar territory in many respects—truth, denial, or undecidability—issues that child protection workers and the courts struggle with every day. But in the period under discussion, the emergent claims in relation to both child sexual abuse and Satanic abuse were projected across the boundary of the professional practice system, beyond the remit of local judicial procedure or media debate, and were then subject to processes of very public national media, legal, and research scrutiny. The Cleveland Inquiry itself, chaired by Justice Butler-Sloss, was obliged to engage at points with the deep philosophical issues to which I have alluded: what kind of thing actually exists in this area, and how secure are our knowledge claims in relation to these phenomena—questions that philosophers would call "ontological" and "epistemological", respectively. Satanic abuse was the subject of the commissioned and careful research study by, interestingly, a distinguished social anthropologist, Jean la Fontaine, who was in effect asked to settle similar questions—do these alleged phenomena exist, and what evidence supports the conclusions reached?

To establish and create social acceptance of new and disturbing social facts of this kind, and to arbitrate conclusively on the status of some closely related social fantasies, are considerable social achievements—assuming the correct judgements were reached. The next phase of public engagement with these issues was perhaps more concerned with meaning and its relationship to historical truth and/or fantasy.

(c) Recovered memory

Debate about "recovered memories" of abuse surfaced in association with the events just recounted, as a kind of third phase of social engagement with the whole terrain. Historical details differ in different

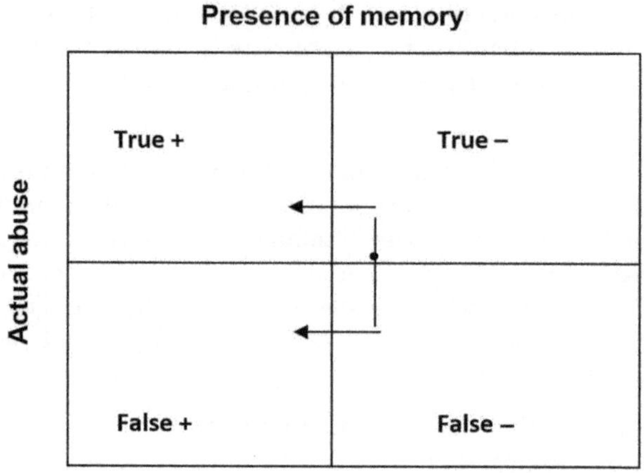

FIGURE 8.2. The relationship between true/false memories and "actual abuse".

countries, and the North American narrative varies from Britain, but in the latter the trajectory is roughly: Cleveland 1987–88, Satanic abuse 1990–1991, recovered memory 1992–5, with a significant conference on the subject organized by the Psychoanalysis Unit at University College London in 1994. The conceptual complexity of the recovered-memory terrain is quite well summarized in Figure 8.2, taken from a chapter of the book reporting the proceedings of that conference:

> Before the recovery (of memory) we do not know whether there was or was not genuine abuse historically, so the supposedly unrecovered information is placed in a neutral position between a false negative and a true negative. The decision is what status to assign to it when it becomes described by the accuser as a genuine memory: is it a true-positive memory or a false-positive memory? The crux of the argument is that the accusers and their therapists are claiming that a false negative becomes a true positive, whereas the False Memory Society parents—who insist on their innocence—are claiming that a true negative becomes a false positive. Both parties can be, and we must assume usually *are*, absolutely sincere. We cannot settle the matter by a show of hands, or even by a lie detector. [Weiskrantz, 1997, p. 6]

Drawing on psychological research into memory and memory recall, the same author concluded that "retrospective analysis of memory in relation to historical events without external corroboration is forever doomed to an uncertain conclusion" (1997, p. 21) and a psychoanalyst commenting on Weiskrantz's chapter remarked that "Perhaps this is one of the hardest things for us—dealing with uncertainty, with having to tolerate not knowing, and not being able to clarify" (Trowell, 1997, p. 25).

But the personal stakes are high, and people pursued certainty in many individual cases through the courts. In her book *Hystories: Hysterical Epidemics and Modern culture*, Elaine Showalter tells us that:

> By 1994 over three hundred cases involving repressed memory had been filed in the American courts. George Franklin was convicted of murder in 1990 and sentenced to life imprisonment when his daughter Eileen "remembered" seeing him kill a child in 1969—a conviction overturned five years later when [the Judge] cited improprieties in the trial and the scientific problems of recovered memory evidence. [Showalter, 1997, p. 146]

Once again, we are in territory broadly defined by the parameters of truth, denial, absolute or partial undecidability, and the tolerance or intolerance of uncertainty. Given this, it is something of a paradox in my account that all of the specific categories of controversy I have so far cited—child sexual abuse, Satanic ritual abuse, and the so-called memory wars that began with recovered memories of abuse—have largely subsided as a focus of public or, indeed, significant professional preoccupation. We accept the reality of, and continue the journey of individual and collective disclosure with respect to, child sexual abuse. I am unaware of Satanic abuse as an element in any case coming to professional attention for many years, and the problem of memory and its relation to historical "truth" has receded into the sequestered space of the consulting room where possibly we are all a little wiser for the intense contestation that occurred. On the other hand, intermittent public turmoil persists concerning those child abuse cases in which there is little or no ambiguity involved, because the child is dead, murdered, often following terrible torture.

Put like this, it does not seem surprising that child abuse and protection become a focus of public concern from time to time. But it is the "time to time" aspect of it that is in part perplexing. The most obvious, and widely accepted explanation for oscillation between public and media indifference, and intense but short-lived concern, is what could be termed the "failure" hypothesis.

Eruptions of public and media concern occur because, and only because, evidence of professional failures to prevent the preventable in these cases come to light. This is complicated territory—we know that in Britain about fifty children a year die at the hands of their parents or immediate carers, and that many of these cases involve what could readily be (re)constructed as "professional failures", the now-familiar recounting of "missed opportunities" to intervene. But year on year, these cases, let alone the many more where children are severely injured, attract little or no pubic or national media attention. No "crisis" ensues. Equally, other public services make mistakes that result in avoidable death—they even seek out and kill innocent people—but entire professions are not vilified in the public mind as a result. Who has heard of police officers or doctors (completely unassociated with the events in question) being spat at in the street or, where they are associated, named and shamed on the front pages of national newspapers?

So, it is tempting to think that the repetitious character of child-death crises in Britain is mostly explained by a toxic blend of an intrusive and scandal-hungry media, a weak social work profession, and occasional instances of egregious and repeated failures to protect vulnerable children. What receives less attention is the idea that these crises are more directly associated with our response to children themselves, and the deaths of particular children, and their terrible suffering at the hands of adults.

(d) Child deaths

There are different points at which the narrative of child murder could be said to begin. I take the series of child deaths in the 1980s that became the subject of high-profile public inquiries as a point of departure: Jasmine Beckford, Kimberley Carlisle, Tyra Henry. Everywhere, in the wake of each of these inquiries, procedures were tightening, volumes of new guidance and procedure being written, risk-assessment protocols drafted. Such was the dominance of this policy response, with which we are now so familiar, that it is hard to imagine it could be different. The story continues through the 1990s and into the twenty-first century: periods of relative calm and re-grouping when the work of child safeguarding professionals is mostly beneath the social radar, punctuated by dramatic eruptions. Each time one of these eruptions occurs, government reacts to public outrage and panic by constructing a further set of rigid procedural or quasi-judicial defences and projecting them back into the professional system, where they are at best ambivalently received but never openly challenged. To a psychotherapist, they appear to be obsessional defences—a lot of ritual checking and re-checking, with an increasing uncertainty about what we are checking *for* (see chapter 4 for a more detailed analysis of obsessional social defences in child protection work).

The obsessional quality of the procedural solutions each inquiry mandates is a reaction characterized, I suggest, by a kind of *excess* rationality, a blind faith in the power of rules to manage and contain the social panic that exposure to the excessively painful and disturbing details of a child murder, and the proximity of someone who might have prevented it but did not, provokes in all of us. Would we have done better, or differently? The thought that we might not have done better is unbearable; the false conviction that we certainly would have done better evokes triumph, rage, and contemptuous dismissal of those who "failed". The result: the now-familiar pronouncement that government will put in place measures to ensure that a dreadful tragedy like this "never happens again".

But it does keep happening—children continue to be murdered, and from time to time news of one of these murders escapes the local professional domain where they are, as it were, routinely if very painfully assimilated, and a further public crisis ensues.

Thus, Figure 8.3 aims to show how recurrently, when controversy and anxiety associated with particular child deaths is propelled out of the realm of the formal child protection system into the public domain (the jagged grey line represents the boundary), the findings and

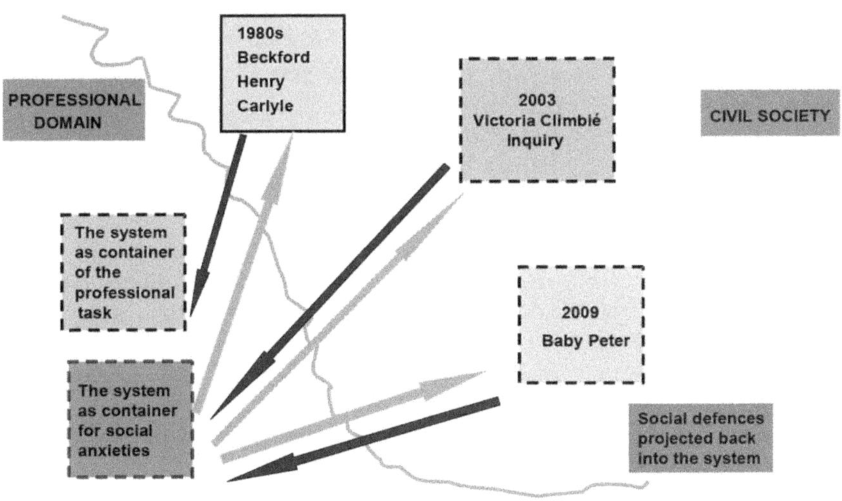

FIGURE 8.3. The recurrent process of reinforcement of defences against child death-related anxieties—from the system to the public sphere and back again.

recommendations of enquiry processes are then propelled back into the official system. The overt task of the system is rendered more difficult, as a result of "failure" in the realm of the "covert" task of protecting the wider public from disturbing awareness and knowledge.

Mourning and its relationship to child death

It was during the Victoria Climbié inquiry that it first occurred to me that the inquiry itself, culminating in the publication of the report, might constitute an unrecognized process of public mourning. To me, it is striking how in every public inquiry process and accompanying media storm, the ordinary emotional registration of the death of the child is lost or is obscured behind the intense preoccupation with questions of blame, accountability, retribution, reconstruction of missed opportunities, and so on. And yet, over the last three decades, the names of perhaps half a dozen of these same children have become inscribed in public memory and discourse, and the (to coin a phrase) often monumentally long and weighty reports of the inquiry into their deaths sit in every academic and many public libraries. Beyond, somewhere out of public reach, are the memories of all the others who died similar deaths but attained no such collective recognition. Like the tomb of the unknown soldier, does each of these inquiries and reports become the one that stands for the many?

In his book *The New Black: Mourning, Melancholia and Depression*, Darian Leader devotes much interesting space to the relationship between public and private mourning. I take this quote as just one of many possible useful points of departure:

> Most Western human beings in fact watch images of death every night in the TV shows about crime scene investigation and murder that fill up the evening programme schedule. It is amazing to realize that this is what most people do after work: they watch programmes in which someone dies and whose death is subsequently explained and made sense of. The fact that this is reiterated endlessly suggests that death is ultimately not something that can be made sense of. And that the increasingly violent images multiply in the absence of a symbolic framework that might mediate them. [Leader, 2009, p. 74]

Do we possess a public symbolic framework to make sense of, to mediate, child murder and torture in our society? I suspect not. The first part of this chapter suggested that each eruption of new awareness in relation to child abuse—Cleveland, Satanic abuse, recovered memories—was succeeded by a process via which public institutions were engaged in an effort at some sort of "sense making", and that these may have been broadly successful. The wearisome and professionally damaging repetition of eruptions over several decades with respect to child deaths suggests something else, but what? Darian Leader takes an observation of Melanie Klein's about internal processes of mourning as the departure point for his discussion of the private–public relationship which he calls "a dialogue of mournings":

> In the mourner's state of mind, the feelings of his internal objects are also sorrowful. In his mind, they share his grief, in the same way as actual kind parents would. The poet tells us that "Nature mourns with the mourner". [Klein, 1940, p. 359]

Contemporary controversies over the phenomenon of public mourning are telling here, says Leader. Critics of, say, the outbreak of public mourning at the death of Diana Princess of Wales, those who characterized the public demonstrations of grief as cynical or inauthentic, are missing the point. "No one really could seriously argue that these tears are [only] for the dead figure themselves. Rather," he says, "it is the public framework that allows people to articulate their own grief for other, unrelated losses. . . . This is a basic function of public mourning rituals. The public facilitates the private" (Leader, 2009, p. 77). On this argument, we could recognize the now-widespread public practice of establishing temporary shrines at the site of a death or loss—road accidents, for example—usually in the form of collections of flowers, as an effort to establish or re-establish a wider public symbolic framework for mourning than private burial rites allow.

Darian Leader explores the many vicissitudes of the mourning process both intrapsychically, and socially, via the anthropology of mourning rituals in various societies. In some societies these rites entail a concrete re-ordering of social relationships in the community "After mourning and burial rites, social structures change, and formal rules govern the new set of ancestors to their descendants. The key is that the dead are installed in the ancestral line." To achieve this, he argues that the dead must be killed a second time. "[F]or the living to feel safe and secure, the dead have to die twice. Real biological death is thus different from proper symbolic death" (2009, p. 116). We might think here both of the impulsive and reactive re-ordering of professional systems that usually follows inquiries, and of the inevitability, as we put it, that "heads will roll" somewhere in those same systems. Only then, at a public level, can the symbolic death *of the child* be secured.

The core thesis I have been outlining in this chapter is that the social history of child abuse in Britain is about a gradual and episodic struggle to accommodate new and disturbing knowledge of ourselves and, along the way, to better delineate reason from unreason. It involves a rather Hegelian idea of social science as the unfolding of society's consciousness of itself. But if, as Leader suggests, we cannot ultimately make sense of actual death, are we condemned forever to repeat the history of our knowledge of child torture and death in the manner of Jasmine Beckford, Victoria Climbié, and Peter Connelly? The view I am tentatively proposing suggests that our monuments to these children are in some respects a symbol of progress—it has taken repeated single cases to achieve it, but on this view no one can any longer doubt it. Child murder keeps happening—but the violent, unpredictable, primitive social processes that attend their installation suggests otherwise. Child murder keeps happening—but only because incompetent professionals take their eye off the ball.

In the closing part of this section of the chapter, I propose that the notion of tragedy is the lost idea that might guide us towards the development of "a symbolic framework that mediates" these eruptions.

Tragedy—the unacceptable face of modernity

Tragedy is an unfashionable idea, perhaps too associated with an attitude of complacency, of passivity, in the face of "fate". It has resonances of an old world, an old social and moral order, from a time before the optimism of reason declared that "there are no accidents", we can subdue our monsters for ever, ensure it never happens again, and in which, as the sociologist Zygmunt Bauman put it, "contingency, accident and fate are deeply *resented*".

> And there are more than enough reasons for the consciousness of mortality to be traumatic. First and foremost, thinking about death defies thought itself . . . reason's power is to be a guide to good choice, but death is not a matter of choice. Death is a scandal, the ultimate humiliation of reason. [Bauman, 1992, pp. 14–15]

Tragic drama has been a key symbolic framework for mediating this fact. But the problem afflicting the great figures of tragic drama is not that their characters are "flawed", but that they do not *know* themselves to be flawed—Lady Macbeth's overweening ambition, Macbeth's propensity to be bullied by her. If redemption arrives, it is in the form of self-knowledge, not the attainment of perfection: "I am a very foolish fond old man", says Lear "and, to deal plainly, I fear I am not in my perfect mind" (*King Lear*, IV.vii). "Nobody dast blame this man. A salesman is got to dream, boy. It comes with the territory", says one character at the graveside of Willy Loman in Arthur Miller's *Death of a Salesman* (Miller, 1958, p. 222). Of course, these reflections bring me to the troubling intersection between an account that seeks to look beyond the surface public discourses and practices that attend such grave matters as the murder of a child, and our social and professional need for those same discourses and practices. We may draw the line at murdering social workers, police officers, or chief executives who are deemed to have failed in the course of their public duty—though an alarming proportion of the population seem inclined not to draw this line—but retrospectively based criticism or critical interrogation of their practices is the norm.

But if nothing resembling the notion of "tragedy" is available to mediate this pressure, the imperative towards production of a retrospective explanatory account that says, "Events *could* or *would* have been otherwise if x had done y" and therefore "x *should* have done y" and so "The world should be otherwise than it is", is irresistible. There is much more to say about this particular, and inadequate, line of epistemological reasoning. For example, it seems to me to substitute a model of social reality as a closed and linear system for one that is open and non-linear and in better accord with lived experience as an unfolding set of possibilities and choices. So here, I find myself in close agreement with Eileen Munro's own analysis of the situation:

> The big problem for society (and consequently for professionals) is establishing a realistic expectation of professionals' ability to predict the future and manage risk of harm to children and young people. Even when it is ascertained that abuse or neglect has occurred, there are difficult decisions to make about whether the parents can be helped to keep children safe from harm or whether the child needs to be removed. Such decisions involve making predictions about likely future harm and so are fallible. It may be judged highly unlikely that the child will be re-abused but low probability events happen.
>
> It is important to be aware how much hindsight distorts our judgment about the predictability of an adverse outcome. Once we know that the outcome was tragic, we look backwards from it and it seems clear which assessments or actions were critical in leading to that outcome. It is then easy to say in amazement "how could they not have seen x?" or "how could they not have realised that x would

lead to y?" Even when we know the evidence on the hindsight bias, it is difficult to shift it; we still look back and over-estimate how visible the signs of danger were. The hindsight bias:

> *"oversimplifies or trivialises the situation confronting the practitioners and masks the processes affecting practitioner behaviour before-the-fact. Hindsight bias blocks our ability to see the deeper story of systematic factors that predictably shape human performance"* (Woods, D. et al., 2010, 15).
>
> [Munro, 2011b, p.18, emphasis in original]

Here I want principally to note that these frameworks of analysis also serve to eradicate the space of loss and mourning, a confrontation with the fact that one kind of event is absolutely outside our control—the certainty of death.

Conclusion

Eileen Munro's series of reports into child protection work in Britain is almost revolutionary, breaking a decades-long mould of bureaucratic, conceptually linear, and essentially positivist public-policy interventions. Her aims went far beyond simply patching up the damaged state of the system and the social work profession following the Peter Connelly crisis, to embrace a fundamental change in cultural and political sensibilities. How successful she will prove to have been in these ambitious aims, it is still too early to adjudicate. The present chapter does not set out to suggest that her analyses are in any way mistaken or misplaced, but it does propose that there are deeper, wider, and more intangible forces at work in our society driving what has seemed like a "repetition compulsion" with respect to chid maltreatment scandal-making, and that we should be prepared for the fact that in British child protection work, history keeps repeating itself, always as tragedy, never as farce.

CHAPTER NINE

The shock of the real: psychoanalysis, modernity, survival

Introduction

> "If you always do what you always did you always get what you always got."
>
> Anon.

The worldwide "crisis" of psychoanalysis is a crisis in its relationship to late modernity, or post-modernity, which it also helped to produce. I fear that on reading this sentence many psychoanalytic practitioners will switch off and read no further. I hope they will persist. A weakness in most psychoanalytic organizations, and in many practitioners, is a reluctance to see that our organizations are *social* institutions, affected by the same currents of social change and development as the rest of society.

Because of the unique and unusual project that they and their members are engaged with, psychoanalytic institutions are also distinctive, particular, and in certain respects unique kinds of organization. But

An earlier version of this chapter was published as A. Cooper & J. Lousada, "The Shock of the Real: Psychoanalysis, Modernity, Survival", in A. Lemma & M. Patrick (Eds.), *Off the Couch: Contemporary Psychoanalytic Applications* (London: Routledge, 2010), pp. 33–45.

when it comes to navigating change in modern society, such uncritical belief in organizational and professional uniqueness is as much of a danger as it is a necessity. Many psychoanalytic thinkers and practitioners hold that their theory and practice is rooted in truths that are timeless, universal, or at least invariant—and thus indifferent at some level to social and cultural change. So, how are profound change and timeless truth related, or, more pertinently, how are contemporary psychoanalytic institutions coping with this tension?

In this chapter, I discuss the distinctive task that psychoanalytic institutions, and perhaps the whole social institution of psychoanalysis, have in managing change. I suggest, first, that the very nature of the psychoanalytic "project" produces an *excessive* preoccupation with questions of tradition, hierarchy, and authority. I call this the "vertical" dimension of the problem. In turn, these preoccupations make it harder to respond realistically to, and to take seriously, the challenges and changes posed by the social environment in which psychoanalysis now operates. Other therapies with their own traditions have grown up, flourished, and may be completely uninterested in psychoanalysis' preoccupation with itself and its traditions. These same therapies are now challenging psychoanalysis within the late modern "free" market of ideas and practices. How do psychoanalytic institutions seem to be responding? I call this the "lateral" dimension of the problem.

A melancholic voice of tradition

The distinctive and unique character of the psychoanalytic project, and one of the characteristic ways in which psychoanalysis defends itself against the threat posed by the contemporary environment, was illustrated for me when a colleague and I gave an early version of this chapter as a paper to an institute of psychoanalytic psychotherapy in Britain. The paper did issue a clear challenge to the audience, which might be summarized as, "See yourselves as others might see you: just another therapeutic institution. So, engage with the new rivals, or risk isolation and death." The second or third speaker from the audience then made the following intervention. She said:

> "Some years ago, shortly before he died, I had the great privilege of having clinical supervision with Dr A (a well-known senior psychoanalyst), and something he often impressed upon me was this—'never forget the unconscious'."

I think that direct engagement with the unconscious is *the* defining feature of psychoanalysis, and that from it flow most of our strengths and joys, but also most of our woes and tribulations. It was only afterwards that we realized how this speaker had both reminded everyone of the core of what psychoanalytic practitioners are fighting to preserve and, simultaneously (and we think unconsciously!), disabled any capacity in the meeting to think new thoughts about the problems facing us. The speaker (a senior member of a psychotherapy institute) evoked the image of a revered, perhaps idealized, but definitely dead psychoanalyst; the sense was of a master at whose feet she had been privileged to learn, and of his voice admonishing us from beyond the grave with a message that says something like, "Do not forget or betray your central vows . . .".

In retrospect, it seemed to us that this was a melancholic voice of tradition and authority, making its appearance to remind us all not to stray from the true path, whatever that may be. It is not a voice that says, "You may have learned much from me, but I am now dead. You must now think your own thoughts, live your own life, find your own path—for being dead, I can know nothing of the dangers you may now face." In melancholia the loved object has not been relinquished so that psychological development can continue, or resume, following profound loss. The unmourned lost love is not available as a source of internal strength but persists as a kind of memorial, transfixing us in relation to the past. Now, more than ever, as it faces new and unprecedented challenges, I propose that psychoanalysis as an institution must have the strength to mourn so that it can simultaneously value its own history and origins.

Slaves of a master discourse?

A central problem faced by psychoanalytic institutes and practitioners is the deep-rooted assumption that psychoanalysis is a "master discourse". This assumption may have been justified in some respects for many decades, but no longer. The slaves have been freed, or have freed themselves. They are now entitled and feel themselves entitled to vote—and even to elect presidents. If this metaphor has resonance, then the history of some societies in which enslaved or systematically oppressed peoples have been liberated might give psychoanalysis realistic cause for concern. How will the slave treat the master now? The particular anxieties faced by psychoanalysis in the contemporary period do not, therefore, derive only from questions of how to "negotiate difference and plurality"—though, to be sure, that is part of the picture as we take up our positions on the more "level playing field" of modern civil society—but also from the more discomforting anxieties of guilt and narcissistic injury in facing a history of, if not dictatorship and oppression towards other psychological practices, then certainly hubris and arrogance.

The culturally arrogant face of psychoanalysis is a cliché, but a cliché with a kernel of meaning and truth that psychoanalysis has always found it hard to examine. Is it simply that the institutions and practices of psychoanalysis have usually been part of the cultural establishment, drawing their membership from the same social milieu? Or is something deeper, more psychically "trans-historical", involved? I believe it is, and that it takes the following form. The possibility of psychoanalysis depends upon an act of extraordinary trust. One person agrees to lie down and reveal all that is in his or her mind to someone he or she does not know who sits out of sight and reveals very little at all. This basic structure *is* necessary, and pretty much all attempts to modify it are, in my view, efforts to evade the extreme anxiety it provokes (or should provoke) in both patient and analyst. For surely there is nobody who, on agreeing to enter into the role of patient, does not feel intensely vulnerable to the psychic gaze of the invisible analyst? Defences against this vulnerability may abound, but the core experience is always present. Whether one thinks in terms of idealization or persecution, of ego-ideal or superego, straightaway the central preoccupation is with a powerful, imposing, and always potentially judging other. There is a paradox at the core of the treatment situation: the conditions required to enable the alleviation of mental suffering can and do amplify anxiety in the patient. I suggest that this excessive preoccupation with the psychic "hierarchy" of potency, judgement, and vulnerable dependency never departs the psychoanalytic scene.

In an inspired paper, Warren Coleman (2006) has charted the havoc that the "analytic super-ego" can wreak upon our own psychoanalytic institutions. In a similar vein to this chapter, Coleman says (2006), "I suggest that the leading anxiety in psychoanalytic work is a fear of helplessness, especially being powerless to heal the patient's distress" (p. 101). Citing Kenneth Eissold (1994), he continues:

> . . . since being "well analysed" is an important criterion of professional acceptance and respect, analysts always feel vulnerable in the eyes of their colleagues to the most intimate *ad hominem* arguments. A vicious circle maybe created whereby feelings of anxiety, guilt and

> inadequacy that are an inevitable concomitant of psychoanalytic work are felt to be personal failings that may be pointed out and held against them by colleagues, thus generating further feelings of anxiety, guilt and inadequacy. [Coleman, 2006, p. 100]

Coleman goes on to describe how psychoanalytic institutions generate hierarchies among themselves:

> Put briefly, the analysts train the psychoanalytic psychotherapists and the psychoanalytic psychotherapists train the psychodynamic counsellors. It is therefore no surprise to find among the latter group the greatest persecutory anxiety and the most rigid beliefs about analytic rules and boundaries for it is here that the greatest distance between analytic ideal and clinical reality is to be found. [2006, p. 111]

In effect, part of Coleman's thesis is that the "psychoanalysts" depend for their continuing self-esteem and hierarchical dominance upon being able to successfully project inferiority or weakness into psychoanalytic psychotherapists, who in turn do the same to the "counsellors". But the projections also operate both ways, since the supposedly persecuted groups may fiercely criticize the "analytic arrogance" of the supposedly dominant ones (2006, p. 100).

In Britain in the early decades of the twenty-first century, this projective organization, which has all the hallmarks of a social system functioning as a defence against anxiety (Menzies, 1959), is breaking down. Many counselling trainings, whether psychodynamic or not, could not give a hoot about the British Psychoanalytical Society, or what its members might say or think. Psychoanalytic institutions and clinical services are everywhere challenged by the suddenly emergent confidence of other treatment modalities and, in some cases, their immeasurably greater skill and application in playing at the politics of evidence-based therapies. All varieties of psychoanalytic training and practice have struggled to come to terms with this new state of affairs. They have done so because, over-preoccupied with their own place in a closed hierarchical system of social and organizational relations—the vertical dimension of the problem—they have lacked the means with which to see and respond to what was happening around them in a reality-based fashion.

The development of relationships to the very much enlarged sibling group with whom there is now a continual scrap for recognition and resources—the lateral dimension of the predicament—has been retarded by the preoccupation with "excess hierarchy". The fact is that in most psychoanalytic institutions in Britain there are not enough trainees, not enough patients to treat (so a greater proportion of patients are trainees), and a visible sense of ageing organizations whose dying and retiring membership is not being replenished. In a curious and discomforting conjuncture, the continued assumption of automatic privilege in this rivalrous arena often coexists with frantic anxiety about survival. Thus, a central question becomes, "Can these healers heal themselves—can the same institutions that have given us the means to 'psychoanalyse' organizations and systems of social relationships make use of these potent tools to address their own predicaments?"

Psychoanalytic reflexivity

Against the backdrop of this analysis, I want to describe some experiences of how psychoanalysis has tried to engage with its own conditions of existence as it traverses a period of profound change. These illustrations are all based in my own experience and work, and they take as their object our own organizational and social experience as a psychoanalytically informed "change agent" in relation to psychoanalytic institutions. This is what is sometimes called "reflexivity"—a variety of "thinking about thinking" that is not solipsistic, because it also engages with thought about reality in some tangible form. Countertransference work is a form of reflexivity, as the analyst thinks about his or her emotional experience and tries to elucidate who has made what contribution to the production of a directly apprehended state of mind. A clinical interpretation rooted in countertransference reflection is an *intervention* in the psychic field produced by patient and analyst with the aim of promoting understanding and, possibly, psychic change. Likewise, the work discussed in this chapter, and the chapter itself, are intended to be interventions in the psychoanalytic cultural and social field.

An aspect of the cultural arrogance of psychoanalysis already mentioned is seen whenever a clinician or theorist deploys psychoanalysis with the aim of "analysing the other" (be it patient, colleague, organization, social process) from a superordinate stance implying privileged access to the unconscious of the other; the assumption of such access in turn justifies the epistemological and moral right to adopt the superordinate stance. This manoeuvre, in which the other is "positioned" as a "*sujet qui est supposé de ne pas savoir*" is the precise antithesis of reflexivity, but often masquerades as it.

A training in psychoanalytic method *does,* however, confer the advantage of skill or capacity to recognize and make sense of unconscious process and communication. As Bion (1994) observed, "It is important to recognize that there is a world in which it is impossible to see what a psycho-analyst can see, although it may be possible for some of those who come for analysis to realize that we see certain things which the rest of the world doesn't see" (p. 319). However, this is *just* a rather unusual kind of skill and in no way justifies the adoption of a morally superior stance. A good plumber or electrician knows things that most of us do not, but we are justifiably irritated if he or she adopts an attitude, as the occasional one does, of moral superiority towards us on the basis of our ignorance. The task at hand is to hold on to what we *do* know, and know about, while coming to terms with a world that accords psychoanalysis less automatic deference than it once did. Resolving how to cope with the collapse of a claim to "master-discourse" status, while avoiding the false solutions offered by notions of patient–clinician democracy or co-construction of the therapeutic process, is a further translation of the contemporary psychoanalytic predicament that is the subject of this chapter.

In the realm of social or political analysis, the attitude of psychoanalytic moral superiority towards the other often takes the form of a complaint in which "they"—often those holding political power or influence—are derided for their lack of psychological sophistication or appreciation of the irrational dimensions of the political process. Of course, this is all too often an accurate depiction. But the important question is the spirit in which this "interpretation" is proffered: is it one that invites dialogue and engagement, or is it one that subtly denigrates the political class for their stupidity and concreteness? At the risk of myself committing the sin of psychoanalytic arrogance against psychoanalysis, it seems to me that the latter is nothing but a variety of narcissistic defence in which intellectual and moral superiority is reasserted in the face of a threatening and powerful other, and the anxieties of engagement and dialogue with this other are evaded.

Changing states of mind

What are the important features of the social world of early twenty-first-century Britain? What should psychoanalytic institutions and their leaders know if they are to facilitate a place for psychoanalysis within it?

First, it is a world in which the relationship between "representation" and "reality" has altered irrevocably, so that we can no longer so confidently assert the epistemological or ontological priority of the latter over the former. It always was possible to "play" with their relationship—for example, to produce "art", or to deceive, con, and manipulate oneself or others—and, of course, in psychoanalytic understanding, creativity and perversion are closely related (Chasseguet-Smirgel, 1985). But in the old world if we "suspended disbelief" during an evening at the theatre or pursued a course of treacherous action, we also knew, or believed we knew, how to rediscover or reassert the psychological or moral *terra firma* we had departed from. It is now somewhat less certain that this is the case.

The British welfare state, including the NHS and personal social services, were forged in a spirit of moral certainty and practical realism—the alleviation of poverty, ignorance, disease, unemployment, and homelessness—that reflected this modernist or enlightenment commitment to the possibility of intervening in human affairs on the basis of good scientific and social-scientific knowledge. State provision of mental health services formed a part of this project, even if it always was too small and undervalued a part. For a time, psychoanalysis also played an influential, though never dominant, part in this practical vision. The Tavistock and Portman clinics, the psychiatric social work profession, and the work of voluntary organizations like the Family Welfare Association established a solid and respected place at the heart of the inevitably contested terrain of understanding and treatment of mental health difficulties.

If psychoanalysis found an automatic niche within this world, it is because the welfare state enacted certain dominant assumptions of the late modern period—faith in science, rationality, and humane projects of social improvement. Applied psychoanalysis was part of the grand inheritance of the modernist project that Marx, Darwin, and Freud bequeathed us. Even if most psychoanalytic psychotherapy in Britain was conducted outside this milieu in private practice, the public/private boundary always was a defining and controversial marker. Patients and therapists travelled across this boundary, or not, and much depended upon the relative resourcing of both individuals and institutions situated either side of this divide. The relative simplicity of this social geography was not to last.

The logic of "state provision" and the logic of "state-funded provision" are completely different; the logic of the nation state and of the market are equally different. Of course, as the state has retreated and, via the introduction of market mechanisms, reconfigured its role in relation to the rest of society, much of the political history of the last decade has been devoted to convincing us otherwise. The market relationships that are now integral to the functioning of the NHS, social services, and the whole public sector in Britain are not those of the so-called perfect or free market, but their radical qualitative impact on the nature of mental health work, child care work, and so on is not diminished because of this. In this world, considerations of cost, efficiency, and effectiveness combine with "rational" managerial principles to produce a context that continually strives to appear to be the best of all known worlds. In the competition to produce evidence for treatments or interventions, those that have done the best job of playing the scientific game can and do present themselves as "*the* best". Branding, marketing, management, cost, efficiency, and public legitimation through science move in *alongside* traditionally grounded truth claims about what might really be the best treatment for a particular condition.

Often, the resulting commodification of psychotherapy is much bemoaned by psychotherapists. But let us not forget that commodities *can* do well in markets, in part at least *because* of their inherent qualities. To forget this is to fall prey to a splitting process in which the good old world that valued truth and reality has been overwhelmed by the bad new one in which relativism and appearances have swept all before them. Equally, however, very good commodities have disappeared without trace from the market because they lost out in the beauty competition of appearances. If this seems like an unfair and irrational way to organize human services in our society, we would not dispute the judgement. But how well did psychoanalysis listen when competitor therapies complained of the unfair hegemony of a world in which psychoanalysis just took its privileged place for granted? Was this a just, fair, and rational way to organize matters?

In our book *Borderline Welfare: Feeling and Fear of Feeling in Modern Welfare* (Cooper & Lousada, 2005), we tried to chart our own and others' experience of the complex and painful transition the British welfare state and public sector has made over the last twenty years from one kind of world to another. Arguably, the old welfare state, and the individual practices it encouraged, was modelled on a metaphor that is instantly recognizable within psychoanalytic discourse: the provision of good, unconditional care and attention to the ill, unhappy, distressed, lost, conflicted, needy self of the patient or client. If this metaphor has lost much of its resonance, this is because it has been purposefully elbowed aside to make room for a new one: that of the rational, strategic, calculating consumer of opportunity in the market place of health and welfare choice. In subsequent work we looked at the more objective political and policy conditions that explain the hold this metaphor has had for recent governments. But however one views the modern British state and its relationship to civil society, it is a different animal from the one that most "senior" figures in our psychotherapy institutes grew up with. Younger members of our society are different too—less deferential, more questioning, more strategic, choosier perhaps. They are by no means pure "consumers" of rational-choice economic theory and, as all the research evidence indicates, not necessarily "happier", but if anything they are probably less persuaded than previous generations that psychoanalysis or its close relatives offer any answers.

In this climate, what is the task facing psychoanalysis and its associated practices? I suggest it is confidently to reassert its commitment to what might be called epistemological realism—a doctrine in which human suffering, mental pain, and unconscious experience are understood to be real, knowable phenomena with direct material effects on personal and social life—while also accepting a more modest, contributory position than hitherto in the much more open, fluid, and contested field of ideas and practices that constitute our late modern cultural milieu.

And minds of state . . .

What does the theory and practice of psychoanalytic psychotherapy have to do with freedom? Are the contemporary challenges facing psychoanalysis a threat to the pursuit of human freedom, which its practices are deemed to embody? The twenty-first-century context of professional regulation for the psychotherapy professions, itself a reflection of the wider direction of "market-state" travel, creates a sharp division in responses to these questions. On the one hand are those who hold that the "stranglehold" of state bureaucracy is a direct threat to the inalienable freedoms of the consulting room; on the other are those who hold that psychoanalysis and its associated therapies are unique contributors to the project of sustaining a socially organized response to mental pain, trauma, and the intergenerational transmission of psychic damage. As Michael Rustin has said:

> . . . the idea that mental pain and anxiety constitute valid claims on social attention has import for broader principles of social organization, qualifying and constraining the logic of markets or bureaucracies as arbiters of social life.
>
> . . . It seems that different perspectives on unconscious aspects of mental life give rise to different political and social outlooks. Outright denial of the existence of the unconscious domain within the behaviourist psychological tradition typically generates interest-based and coercive models of social organization. Insistence, by contrast, on the repressive aspects of all symbolized social order generates a countervailing politics of resistance and "subversion", tending to demand the revolutionary overthrow of the "authoritarian symbolic" . . . [M. J. Rustin, 1995, p. 241]

Psychoanalysis has always had a number of "radical" wings, though none of them can be complacent about their ability to have freed themselves from the illness of cultural arrogance discussed earlier. Rustin is pointing out the relationship between different conceptions of the psychoanalytic project (and of the unconscious) and the very different political strategies that tend to flow from these, including *strategies for the institutions of psychoanalysis itself* within processes of social change. In Britain today, those who support the project of professional regulation for psychoanalytic psychotherapy, which is to say the incorporation of psychoanalytic psychotherapy within the confines of state scrutiny, legitimation, inspection, and so on, may have many well-founded anxieties about the potential for external bureaucratic impingements. However, the leading umbrella organization for psychoanalytic psychotherapy, the British Psychoanalytic Council (BPC, 2008a, 2008b), while supporting regulation, has also positioned itself clearly within a psychoanalytic tradition of radical *social* provision, first outlined by Freud himself:

> At present we can do nothing for the wider social strata, who suffer extremely seriously from the neuroses. . . . [T]he poor man should have just as much right to assistance for his mind as he now has to the life-saving help offered by surgery . . . out-patient clinics will be started to which analytically trained physicians will be appointed. [Freud, 1919a, p. 167]

From this starting point, the only important question is whether a political position inside the apparatus of state regulation, or even a position "in and against" this state apparatus, constitutes a viable site of struggle towards greater "positive" freedoms for the general population who need access to highly trained, and responsible, psychoanalytic clinicians. Set against this perspective, the objections of some to the feared intrusion of regulatory principles into the free-associative space in which psychoanalytic psychotherapy takes place appear abstract, philosophically self-indulgent, and individualist. The struggle for psychic freedom and the struggle for social and political freedom are linked—and both occur under conditions of inevitable and necessary constraint. Psychoanalysis never conceived of itself (except in certain romantic appropriations) as a practice that could or would promise deliverance into a world of absolute freedom—Freud and every major subsequent psychoanalytic theorist are at one with the spirit of Karl Marx's thought here: men make their own history, but not under conditions of their own choosing.

Of course, it is possible that the British state bureaucratic machine will develop in a direction that requires from psychoanalysis a different, more politically challenging response. But like all judgements about political action, this is one that depends upon the "material conditions" that pertain at any point in time. How bad does it have to be before psychotherapists take up arms against the state? In one sense, no one can answer this question before it happens. But before even contemplating the answer, one might consider all the evidence we already do have for the link between mental pain and social conditions that both the state *and* psychotherapists continually "forget". This knowledge is the ground on which a real psycho-political struggle—with huge and real potential benefits for the population—could *now* be fought, if only both parties were not complicit in this defence of forgetting. The following are some of the salient facts.

High-quality research conducted over many years in many countries convincingly shows that the prevalence of mental health problems in any one country is directly correlated with the level of income inequality in that country—that is to say, a measure of how much more is earned by the richest one-fifth of the population, compared to the poorest fifth (Wilkinson & Pickett, 2009). Many other measures of social and personal distress and dysfunction are similarly correlated with income inequality. As it happens, Britain emerges rather badly from this particular set of league tables simply because, assessed by this criterion, it is one of the most unequal countries in the developed world.

Research conducted some decades ago into the "social origins" of depression (Brown & Harris, 1978) showed how the prevalence of clinical depression among women is significantly a function of social class, mediated by a specific group of "vulnerability factors" that, in the presence of significant adverse life events (but not without these), trigger depression. Some of these "vulnerability factors" (such as the loss of the subject's mother in childhood) point towards the importance of causal factors that are familiar to psychoanalytic psychotherapists. But many of the significant causal variables in this study are not straightforwardly psychological or intrapsychic. Wilkinson and Pickett are interested not just in the correlations they have unearthed, but in the explanatory mechanisms that might link social inequality with, for example, a history of mental health problems.

But how interested are most psychoanalytic psychotherapists in these perspectives? How do they account for the powerful explanatory force of findings such as these, and the seemingly radical disjunction with traditional psychoanalytic theory they imply? According to these other perspectives, mental health and illness seem, at a minimum, to be psycho-social phenomena even if not "political" ones—though the link with material inequalities makes it hard to avoid this latter suggestion. If this is so, and psychotherapists are treating the same, or similar, people who are the research subjects in these studies, surely the question must arise: "What are the right forms of practical and moral engagement of the psychoanalytic psychotherapist *as psychotherapist* with the society in which she or he practises? Can the psychotherapist and the citizen or political subject be uncoupled one from the other?"

Conclusion

Does the psychodynamic counsellor have anything to teach the psychoanalyst about the practice of therapy? Does the psychodynamic counsellor have anything to teach the analyst about the nature of unconscious processes?

The questions are designed to disturb—to disrupt some taken-for-granted assumptions about professional and training hierarchies that for too long have organized the internal and external world of psychoanalysis and psychotherapy in this country. To secure its future in the late modern, twenty-first-century marketized world, psychoanalysis must learn to travel "more lightly", to free itself from any melancholic attachment to its founders, from the need to maintain hierarchies of privilege and status rather than those of meaning and expertise. These "vertical" and "lateral" dimensions of the problem facing psychoanalysis are intertwined with many other antinomies that require a more fluid engagement: the pure and the applied, the public and private, the ancient and the modern, the professional and the political, and so forth.

To recapitulate: as a psychoanalytic psychotherapist, how one engages with the public or social sphere may depend very significantly on how, at root, one frames the task of psychoanalytic therapy itself. Is it primarily a treatment for mental pain and distress, or is it primarily a method for investigating and learning about unconscious processes? These are not the only possible alternatives, nor are they absolutely mutually exclusive ones, but maybe they do help us to bring into focus the very different and not always explicit self-images and images of others that we deploy. If psychoanalytic psychotherapy is primarily a treatment for mental pain, then the question "Can a psychodynamic counsellor have anything to teach a psychoanalyst" will seem neither surprising nor contradictory: many psychodynamic counsellors work in public and publicly funded settings with populations that are unlikely ever to access psychoanalysis. How to work effectively in once-weekly short-term treatments, or how to consult effectively to hard-pressed GPs or Practice Nurses are among the many matters that counsellors may be better equipped to tackle and advise upon than is a psychoanalyst in full-time private practice. In the complex, messy world of front-line mental health services, the psychoanalyst can lay claim to very few privileges, in my view.

But if psychoanalysis or psychoanalytic work of any kind is only possible on the basis of a sophisticated appreciation of unconscious processes, then here the traditional remit of the psychoanalyst must surely reign. Working analytically at five-times-a-week intensity over many years constitutes the privileged "laboratory conditions" for experiencing, elucidating, and theorizing the nature of the unconscious and the complex configurations of desire, defence, history, and possibility that is human development. This is the same work that Freud himself began, and the same work that underpinned his radical call for psychoanalysis to be widely available as a response to both personal and social afflictions.

We must avoid the temptations of elitism so often associated with the project of "pure science" while preserving our capacity to nurture excellence; equally we must embrace the potential for psychoanalytically informed therapy to be popularized and made widely available without consigning this to an inferior realm of the "applied". This chapter is intended to be a contribution to helping us manage these tensions in an open and undefensive fashion. The survival of psychoanalysis may depend on this.

CHAPTER TEN

Containing tensions: psychoanalysis and modern policymaking

What can contemporary psychoanalysis offer to modern policymaking and progressive political practice? Psychoanalysis today offers a distinct vision for politics, bringing learning from the dyadic encounter between therapist and patient and from interventions across the strata of society. It posits that there is an urgent need for emotionally intelligent policymaking, which grapples with and roots itself in the complex realities of social relations and forges negotiated solutions. We have become used to rational-linear, "top-down" policymaking, but such processes fail to contend with the messy and often conflictual systems and domains in which we live, where our fears, desires, and agonies inevitably play a role. Modern psychoanalysis asks that policy thinking uses this understanding of society as a departure point for theory and action.

At a time when neoliberalism is the dominant ideology, psychoanalysis today also offers a critique of its reductionist view of human nature. Psychoanalysts daily witness the dehumanizing impact of neoliberal forces on our organizations, relationships, and subjective identities (Cooper & Lousada, 2005; M. J. Rustin, 1991a). This chapter begins with a series of vignettes that trace the pathway between psychoanalytic practice and policy thinking, and between personal experience and social experience.

Among the people

In a disadvantaged inner-city community centre, a multi-ethnic group of residents sit in a circle recounting their painful personal histories, conflicted relationships, struggles with everyday poverty, and helplessness in the face of local bureaucracy. This is a "Thinking Space" (Lowe, 2014), a weekly community therapy project started by a psychoanalytic therapist in the aftermath of the 2011 riots. The therapist facilitates the encounter by listening intently, linking different experiences and contributions, and occasionally commenting on the painfulness of a member's story. This project owes something to the spirit of Paulo Freire's philosophy of "conscientization", first articulated in his *Pedagogy of the Oppressed*, but its founder was drawing on his own experience as a black therapist, concerned to take a psychoanalytic sensibility beyond the clinic and into the messy arena of lived experiences in fractured communities. This work is about developing understanding of social suffering and enabling supportive connections—among people who might never speak to one another but share common predicaments, and between the realm of personal pain and social conditions of disadvantage, racism, and exclusion. Private troubles and public issues (Wright Mills, 1959) come into relationship.

In an East London children's centre, a psychoanalytically trained social worker welcomes a dozen children who arrive in various groupings with their foster carers. The children are members of three sibling groups, all of them in local authority care and in the process of being adopted or placed in long-term foster care. The adoption worker had noticed something that no one else had registered: that large sibling groups are routinely split up when they enter the care system, and then planning for the futures of sub-groups proceeds on separate lines. Professionals "forget" the wider sibling system and cease to consider its meaning from the children's point of view. The series of groups she facilitates brings the sub-groups back into connection and then helps them say goodbye, but now in the context of a system that "remembers" their relationships and will enable future contact. Her work was fiercely resisted at first by her managers, by judges, and by Children's Guardians. They all voiced the same reaction: this process would be too painful for these children, and the work would harm them. But she won them round, helping them discover that this response was mostly about the pain evoked in *them* at the prospect of these meetings and mournings.

A psychoanalytically trained psychologist is consulting to a GP in an inner-city health centre about one of her patients who uses the service frequently, but for whom conventional physical medicine appears not to work. The GP feels useless and helpless but obliged to continue seeing the patient. The patient doesn't get any better but seems adhesively attached to the health centre. Something more is going on, and the consultation aims to understand what and then how best to alleviate the GP's burden while providing the patient some help he can use.

"Containment" is a central concept in modern psychoanalysis, denoting a capacity for emotional receptivity towards other people's psychic and relational conflicts, traumas, and anxieties (sometimes known as the "contained"). The containing faculty promotes psychological growth and maturation by tolerating the turbulence of unspeakable anxiety or conflict, rather than jumping to "problem-solve" it or deny its reality. This is the function that the key actors in the vignettes above are aiming to provide. Successful containment reanimates groups, organizations, and individuals, freeing them from disabling anxiety. It underpins an ability to generate authentic depth in our understanding of social relations, resonating with Jonathan Freedland's (2015) appeal to the Labour Party, in its search for a revitalizing narrative following the election defeat of 2015, to master "an emotional rather than a rational idiom" and to speak in a language people actually use.

The idea of "social containment" and of society as a container has been most fully developed by Barry Richards (2007, 2018) in his work on emotional governance and political leadership. His thinking is closely related to work he and others have developed on the theme of "therapeutic culture" as a relatively recent "expressive" aspect of modern society in which the self is understood, in social context, through the discourses of psychotherapy as these have permeated popular culture and language. Political, media, and commercial relationships with citizens and social groups are increasingly attentive to and constituted by attention to emotional processes. With reference to the nation state as a "containing object", Richards says:

> Overall my hypothesis is that the quasi-parental functions of protective authority and nurturing provision endow the state with powerful unconscious resonance, however distant or alienated from it any individual might feel. In its functions of protector and provider, the state is the actual source of many potentially containing objects in our everyday environment. It is where we turn for defence both

> against those who wish to do us harm, be they antagonistic neighbours, domestic criminals or self-defined enemies on the other side of the world, and against the forces of nature, be they storms, floods, disease or infestation. It is also the producer or the guarantor of the material infrastructure of society, and for most of us it is the primary or sole provider of the life-giving social goods of education and the health and welfare services. [2018, p. 77]

Richards' work on social containment represents a subtle and wide-ranging attempt to "map" the emotional matrices that bind, or not, social relations and societies in their affective dimensions. He is concerned to argue the case for a positive notion of containment as a reality and a possibility. My own approach is slightly different, but complementary, I think, arising as it does from a primary preoccupation with processes and events wherein containing social relationships are manifestly absent, with destructive or unhelpful social and personal consequences. My sense of how containment "works" is also perhaps more clinically grounded, with a close eye to the fine grain of how processes in which intolerable anxieties, and the predicaments of populations who are "out of social mind", cannot be thought about and understood in the absence of a social or professional "apparatus" for symbolizing and representing their meanings. The examples given in the present chapter are one kind of instance, while the explosive and destabilizing processes associated with child protection crises are examined fully in chapter 8, and the containing potential of the present Independent Inquiry into Child Sexual Abuse in chapter 7.

We may associate psychoanalysis with lying on a couch five times a week for years on end, but Freud himself hoped that psychoanalytic practice would lead to the kinds of provision sketched out above. He wrote: "It is possible to foresee that the conscience of society will awake and remind it that the poor man should have just as much right to assistance for his mind as he now has to the life-saving help offered by surgery. . . . Such treatments will be free" (Freud, 1919a). Containment was unavailable to Freud as a concept, clinical or otherwise, but it represents the most significant addition since his time to the armoury of psychoanalytic understanding of social processes.

Deep or shallow welfare?

The adoption worker described above is doing more than just advocating for the needs of a specific group of disadvantaged children. She is doing the work of a "boundary spanner" (Williams, 2002), conveying thickly textured emotional and social intelligence from one domain to another in search of a more attuned and grounded policy response rooted in authentic recognition and understanding of lived experiences. She is insisting that the policy process must begin from such understanding, shape itself around such complex realities, and forge solutions that are negotiated between these different domains and systems. Psychoanalytically, she is asking the social "container" to relate to, incorporate, and digest the quality of experience of the "contained" before it delivers a solution or policy response. She is resisting the baleful impact of what Foucault termed "governmentality", the dominance of expert systems of ordering and control that shape social relationships and subjectivity, especially those populations without "voice", through the medium of policy and bureaucracy. These sibling groups have a better chance of a more connected life when decisions made *about* them by a "container" are decisions forged in dialogue *with* them.

The above vignettes also offer an implicit critique of rational–linear policymaking, echoed in the work of systems theorist Jake Chapman (2004) who argues that governments must learn to "think differently" about the relationship between policy processes and the social realities in which they intervene. The latter can never be fully controlled, and the unanticipated consequences of their independent agency, resistance, or expression of alternative desires inevitably disrupt and distort the best-laid policy plans. Better policymaking means relinquishing some control, and hence power. More meaningful, thickly textured social relations are the gain.

Healthy organizations

The marriage of psychoanalytic and systems thinking in organizational development work is long established. Intensive "Group Relations Events" (GRE), involving up to a hundred participants, are the medium for learning here, not the therapeutic dyad. But the focus is similar: the close study of the interplay of primitive, affective, and irrational forces with rational, structured, task-oriented purposes that produce the messy, conflicted reality that is institutional life. Learning to tolerate and understand the former, in order to detoxify their impact on the latter, is one key objective. Again there are echoes of the "container–contained" relation. People often find they are disproportionately scared in these events and deeply suspicious of the intentions and good faith of the staff. They lose voice and agency as a result, but exploration and working though of these fears enables "recovery".

Groups regain their power to do business with the staff group and negotiate successfully for their aims and projects. The temporary institution of the GRE starts to resemble a participatory democracy, a form of interaction central to the work of therapeutic communities. This is representative of a tradition of mental health work now eviscerated from the NHS, despite evidence of cost effectiveness, and I explored in chapter 5 the resonance of these practices with those of the Tavistock itself.

There is a duality in the application of this work with organizations. One strand emphasizes how the management task must take its lead from a close appreciation of the character of the organization's work (Hutten, Bazalgette, & Armstrong, 1994). One size does not fit all, and each organization has its own particular "under the surface" struggles. Managing a care home for vulnerable and dying people is not the same as managing an airport. The existential anxieties of "living with dying" as a day job may give rise to protective behaviours in staff that mitigate against the provision of close emotional attention to residents. Close analysis of an airport's "task" discloses it to be all about "flows" and disruptions of flow—passengers, baggage, planes, weather conditions, with disruptions in Hong Kong or Paris affecting London or Manchester. Our need for predictable, stable conditions in which to work and live is fundamental, but tolerance of instability and confusion as normal is a requirement for the airport manager. The emotional capacities required of staff in each context are particular, but the tendency to protect against their discomforting aspects with anti-task behaviours is similar.

Thus the study of "social systems as a defence against anxiety" is the complimentary contribution of psychoanalysis to institutional life. Protective strategies against task-related anxiety become inscribed in organizational operating systems, and their normalization disguises their negative impact. Unpicking them exposes everyone to more anxiety, but facilitates a deeper, better connected, and more fulfilling working experience. Recent work in human service organizations (Cooper & Lees, 2014) proposes that the impact of the emotional strain of responsibility for children and adults "at risk" intersects with governmental anxieties about "failure", performance, and standards, to produce a culture of fear in staff and management alike—fear, anxiety, and guilt about doing harm to service users, but also fear for the survival of the self in case of external judgements of incompetence which lead to a perverse focus on meeting targets rather than meeting needs. This climate is not conducive of confident care. Tim Dartington's (2010) work on managing vulnerability then develops a higher order analysis of "heroic" stances in health care, in tension with more "stoical" dispositions in the less prominent but equally vital domain of social care. Neither leaves space for a more tragic perspective that embraces the brute fact of our mortality.

Towards emotionally intelligent policymaking

In 2007, I shared a conference platform with a senior civil servant, just after the government first announced substantial funding for its Improving Access to Psychological Therapies (IAPT) programme. He was heckled by sections of the audience of three hundred therapists of various persuasions, and finally exploded—"You're worse than my grandchildren! What are you complaining about? You've just been given 300 million pounds!" He seemed genuinely baffled. But in the eyes of many, the money had been given to the wrong kind of therapists. Psychoanalytic therapy was excluded from this vision, and to the dissenters CBT had just won an unjustified victory in the scrap for political legitimation. The man's reaction was understandable, but not emotionally intelligent. In an instant he lost the sympathy of half his audience. Had he been better briefed, or had he cared more about the internal tensions in this community, he might have anticipated a partially hostile reception, absorbed it, and there and then done some useful work with it to help heal divisions and to moderate the toxicity of competition and rivalry. His leadership would also have benefited from an appreciation of the value of "containment" as a capacity.

Emotionally intelligent policymaking is an idea whose time is overdue and extends well beyond individual leadership. Episodically, the misleadingly calm surface of our social life is ruptured by violence and conflict. The 2011 riots, the repeated eruptions of public anxiety about different forms of child abuse, and the controversy over the Liverpool end-of-life care policy are linked by the fact that the underlying sources of tension were known about, but were also denied, ignored, or inadequately articulated by those who do "know".

Sometimes our reactive mechanisms work to good effect, but often compound the problem. The 1979 Cleveland Inquiry into child sexual abuse decisively progressed our capacity to embrace dangerous knowledge and our work to combat its sources. We now accept that intra-familial sexual abuse has always been widespread across all social strata and communities, but when it surfaced on a large scale in Cleveland this emerging knowledge was fiercely contested by the media and significant sections of the establishment. The agents of disclosure were systematically scapegoated and their actions deemed a "witch hunt" by the sitting local MP. It took a sensitively chaired major public enquiry to achieve a definitive social and political "settlement" about the reality of this phenomenon. But other public enquiry processes default to accusation and blame and a familiar litany of mindless recommendations. Psychoanalytic practitioners have created and deployed more "containing" methodologies of conflict resolution to great effect in Northern Ireland and on the international stage (Alderdice, 2010; Volkan, 2008). Their practices resonate with the work of Truth and Reconciliation Commissions established in many post-conflict situations. The tensions with which these processes work cannot be wished or legislated away, but they can be attended to. It takes years for communities and professions to recover from outbreaks of social or symbolic violence, but such ruptures can be prevented.

Contemporary psychoanalysis asks that policymakers ground themselves in the complexity of social relations and negotiate solutions based on our lived experience. This means more listening, hearing, digesting, and ultimately validating painful, conflicted, and aggrieved personal and social experience.

Between evidence and policy: the crooked line

The British psychoanalytic community is a contradictory beast. Analysts and therapists mobilized strongly around nuclear disarmament in the 1980s, and today they are active in forging cross-disciplinary understandings about the existential threats posed by climate change, and our ambivalence and denial of these same threats (Weintrobe, 2013). NHS-trained child psychotherapists are rooted in public sector work with traumatized and abused children. But the gravitational pull of private practice has always been fierce, with the psychoanalytic establishment's defence of lengthy individual treatments creating an equal and opposite force (Taylor, 2013). At best, though, the intense focus on "inner-world" dynamics combines with trenchant critique of the dehumanizing impact of neoliberal market forces on our organizations, relationships, and subjective identities.

Recent years have seen a spike in books concerned with the various side-effects of neoliberal policy, which tread familiar ground for psychoanalysis. Wilkinson and Pickett's tour-de-force *The Spirit Level* (2009), which should have revolutionized public policy but is sadly fading into intellectual history, showed how rates of mental illness are rising in the more neoliberal and unequal countries on our planet. Their book lent empirical support to the idea that mental health is "psycho-social", rooted in a complex interplay between individual and family biographies, and socio-economic, gender, and ethnic relations. Brown and Harris's (1978) *Social Origins of Depression* disclosed such mechanisms rigorously, but today their work is largely forgotten. More recently, William Davies' *The Happiness Industry* (2015) has provided a potent critique of the way in which neoliberal thinking has tied itself to positivism to commodify subjectivity and promote an individualist concept of mental health and well-being. On this account, we can "choose happiness", or not, and by this logic—which seems to suit the polices of the current government—our personal suffering becomes our responsibility, and failure to surmount it our fault.

And yet, such books aside and feminism notwithstanding, the Left remains uncomfortable with discourses on feeling, subjectivity, and "interiority". Modern psychoanalysis, rooted in a diversity of modes of practice with groups, organizations, families, individuals, and couples (Taylor, 2013), makes the case that policymaking simply cannot afford to ignore our lived experiences. To do so is to ignore the reality that we are not entirely rational, positive beings who fit into neat policy constructs. Historically, the psychoanalytic community has been slow to advance its ideas and practices—there has never been a "movement" to promote its vision for "human flourishing" and emotionally intelligent policymaking. Psychoanalysis has been too convinced of its status as a master narrative and reluctant to see that its vision of "human flourishing" is under attack from forces emanating from far beyond internecine squabbles among different schools of psychology.

Today, the British Psychoanalytic Council is working with vigour to position the full spectrum of psychoanalytic work in the public domain and to publicize the growing evidence base (www.bpc.org.uk). Evidence for the effectiveness of psychoanalytic therapy for both adults and children is good, but historically our ability to communicate this publicly and politically has been poor. CBT managed its policy and public-understanding campaign far better, and for a period this exacerbated latent rivalries between the different therapeutic modalities. There is much rapprochement now, and potent new forms of integrative psychoanalytically led service are emerging (Hard, Rock, & Stern, 2015). The lessons of all this are simple: there is a crooked line connecting the evidence base and evidence-based policy formation. The intervening variables are politics and ideology, as well as a war of cultures which will always favour some varieties of evidence over others. Wars are never won by reason and argument alone, because power, wealth, status, and the systems of influence sustaining these predominate.

Modern psychoanalysis engages with a vast range of sequestered domains of social reality and insists on "surfacing" them for social and political work and attention. This generates a different culture of political and policy processes from that of traditional discourses of rights, opportunities, or redistribution, one that insists on the thick textures of social and personal suffering, desire, and aspiration as its point of departure for theory and action and points to the inherent value of participatory democracy. This concept of society and social action also challenges the dominance of mechanical metaphors that pervade and construct mainstream-policy discourse. Society is not a machine, but a nested tangle of complex systems in which human desires, fears, hopes, and agonies play a major role. A revitalized progressive politics must embrace all this. There is a long road to travel, but slowly Freud's radical vision for psychoanalysis may be coming in from the cold.

CHAPTER ELEVEN

"Be quiet and listen": thinking differently about social policy

Introduction

> "I am working in a factory. I have been working there for the last five years. When I started my job I did not think it was a factory. It didn't look like a factory, not from the outside and not from the inside."

An experienced qualified social worker opened a presentation about her lived experience of the policy environment she inhabited with these words. Many of the practitioners who follow the programme of work leading up to such presentations begin to realize they have been "professionally depressed", because they have long endured organizational and societal working conditions that they experience as oppressive. They have also learned a kind of "helplessness" in the face of these conditions, exacerbated by their belief that they may be punished by their managers if they speak about their experiences. They have learned to "be quiet and listen". The emergence of this "depression" often signals a shift, so people become angrier and more inclined to challenge their own sense of passivity and helplessness.

This chapter explores the idea that we all "live" social policy all of the time, as commuters, parents, children, citizens, consumers, patients, learners, teachers, neighbours, workers. This experience is not readily available to us without a framework of analysis that reveals its policy-embedded nature. Social policy is not a particularly popular subject among students and practitioners of social work and allied professions. On British qualifying social work programmes, the rather dry and unreflective tradition requiring the study of "social administration"—the history, structure and legislative frameworks shaping the welfare state—has much to answer for. But there is another way to do social policy, and this chapter sketches out a model of policy analysis in which the direct everyday experience of policy actors is the point of departure. In particular, the "emotional experience" of the socially situated subject of policy is assumed to be analytically valid and capable of disclosing dimensions of policy processes that are invisible or marginalized without attention to this experiential register of analysis. Viewed like this, policy processes generate specific "structures of feeling" (Williams, 1993) that inform political, professional, and civic culture, constructing and reconstructing our subjectivity and relationships.

Drawing on a blend of psychoanalytic and systemic theory and practice, and on selected resources in social and political theory, this approach to policy analysis is characterized by a concern to interrogate the relationship between "surface and depth" in policy processes, and between "wholes and parts". Policy discourses commonly represent their objects of analysis—social and economic arrangements affecting the lives and well-being of the population—as inherently unified, conflict-free, and fully amenable to change through rationally planned interventions. Frequently, they seem to behave as though they *are* expressions of a consensual and fully rational "social totality". The analytical effort required to interrogate these productions in terms of what they discursively, epistemologically, emotionally, and politically omit, disallow, disavow, obscure, or "forget" is considerable, if their tendency to construct a natural and inevitable order of things is to be challenged. The idea of a false or misleading concept of a "natural order of things" is what we mean by the word "ideology". Thus this chapter is about engaging critically with ideology, and how ideology gets inside us.

The whole–part and surface–depth metaphors aim to capture a "vertical" and a "lateral" dimension for the interrogation of policy processes, in particular of what is absent from their discourses or registers of social engagement; what is "swept aside" (available to be known or understood, but consigned to some other realm of the social whole from where we have to recover its relevance to the policy process at hand); and what is "swept under the carpet" (suppressed, denied, or otherwise rendered unavailable for symbolic elaboration within policy discourse). These metaphors are intended to resemble the psychoanalytic concepts of splitting and repression, which may be one useful source for grounding the critical project of developing an alternative mode of "doing policy."

Thus, the model developed in this chapter constitutes:

- A distinctive mode of policy analysis that is inherently critical of more conventional rationalist models.
- A psycho-social methodology for interpreting and situating social experience insofar as this experience is generated in and through policy processes.
- A basis for developing alternative and creative policy behaviour and interventions that rescue policy actors and analysts from the dangers of "policy dependency".
- A mode of analysis that reconnects with our lived experience, emotionality, critical faculties, and capacity to assume authority for interpreting and changing aspects of the world in which we live.

Why emotion, why psycho-social?

What contribution to policy analysis does a psycho-social focus on emotion offer? Why is it needed? John Simmonds (personal communication, 2008) has characterized the problem of the relationship between policy process and the "real-world" mess, pain, trauma, confusion, and uncertainty of lived social experience as that of "sanitization". Emotional realities are routinely sanitized by policy discourse, by models of policy analysis, and by policy processes themselves. Sanitization excludes real-world emotionality from *influencing* policymakers and policymaking, and it denies the subjects of policy true *recognition* as people with feelings. The result is a form of social and personal alienation that is damaging to our capacity for social progress. The model of policy analysis advanced in this chapter is a start at rectifying this state of affairs.

Public policy analysis is not a monolithic field of study, but despite a diversity of models and theories the dominant paradigm remains technocratic, rationalist, and instrumental. On the basis of studies of how policy processes actually work, Charles Lindblom, a chief critic of rational decision making in policy and policy analysis, advocated an approach called "the science of muddling through" (Lindblom, 1959).

If real-world processes frequently reveal a muddled and incremental picture of progress towards policy goals, then this is for good reasons; there are absolute limits to the possibility of fully rational, logical planning and decision-making processes in complex societies. However, sound policy methodology does not abandon rationality and analysis; rather, it must also respect the messiness, recalcitrance, and complexity of social processes, and thus the "science" of muddling through is born. The approach is similar to the "mixed-scanning" model developed by the communitarian theorist Amati Etzioni (1967), and the two thinkers had a prolonged critical engagement.

However, while these rather limited and still instrumental critiques do acknowledge the place of "irrational" and unpredictable forces and processes in social life, suggesting the notion of "bounded" rationality as a basis for decision making, emotion, and passion still find no place within their models of policymaking or policy analysis. Surely, this is a strange and puzzling omission? Values *do* enter their analytical picture, but usually only as a variable understood to be guiding decisions in pursuit of specific ends or goals—social "goods". Yet, public policies, and the value positions they embody, are frequently the focus of fierce emotional attachments, passions, and private as well as public conflicts. We need only think of the poll-tax riots, airport expansion, congestion charging, university tuition fees. To an important degree, this omission can be ascribed to a distinction, sometimes tacit and sometimes explicit, between the domains of policy and politics. Politics becomes the legitimate site of passion and contestation, policy of instrumental reason and administration. I was alerted to this on one occasion when I was advised by my boss that a policy seminar I had organized on a topic of current controversy seemed to be "more about politics than policy"! The boss had been contacted by a concerned chief executive from a neighbouring organization who feared the seminar would be a covert effort to criticize his own management.

If public policy *is* the continuation of politics by other means, but passions are to be evacuated from policy in the direction of their "legitimate" site—the formal democratic process—we have the beginnings of an understanding of why there is a modern "crisis" of democracy and participation in formal political processes. Most of what directly affects the lives of citizens as a result of the governments they elect is in fact enacted through "policy" and not the democratic process; yet the dominant paradigms of policy seem to convey the message that these are purely technical or instrumental processes that should require no engagement on our part. Suddenly, the presence or absence of emotion and passion as a dimension of policy processes and analysis assumes considerable *ideological* significance.

In contemporary Britain, passionate public debate and active contestation about political alternatives and futures is now muted. There is no single or simple explanation for this change of climate over the last ten or twenty years, but the stripping away of many of the intermediate institutions of civil society that once constituted the collective "voice" of multiple-interest groups is surely central (Cooper & Lousada, 2005; Hutton, 1996). This development helped pave the way for a contemporary political ethic of consumerist individualism and personal "responsibilization". What was once a social contract in which social collectives—trade unions, professions, democratically led institutions—played a vital negotiative role now looks more like a contract between government and the private individual as consumer of tax-funded services (Cooper, 2008c). But, of course, "the social" in the sense of social relationships has not been dissolved, merely disguised and recast in this new individualistic ideological formation.

Psycho-social theory and analysis descriptively capture the new and complex identities and relationships between individuals, groups, social movements, and the "social totality" that emerge in the unfamiliar "spaces" afforded by these new developments, but they also create the opportunity to question, interrogate, and critique these same developments that constitute our emergent psycho-social conditions of existence. If our passionate and emotional connections to each other, but also to the social institutions of which we are members, are indeed obscured or muted in these new life worlds, emotionally grounded psycho-social analysis can return them to us, and us to them.

Be quiet and listen

The thinking in this chapter is partly informed by the experience of the Tavistock Policy Seminars, started in 2004, subtitled "Reconnecting Public Policy and Human Relationships". These seminars run to a simple but effective format that models something of this aspiration to "reconnect" policy processes and emotionally charged social relationships. Two speakers present their perspectives on the seminar theme, usually but not always involving some degree of tension or difference of stance. After a break, the discussion is thrown open to the floor, and the speakers are asked not to contribute until invited to do so towards the end of the event. This requires the audience to relinquish the familiar pattern of questioning the speakers, agreeing with or opposing them in a binary fashion; rather, they are invited to assume responsibility for developing a dialogue among themselves, but in connection with the material presented by the speakers. In turn, it requires speakers to relinquish the expert role—to be quiet and listen. Over the course of an hour, complex, layered thinking evolves that contrasts with the familiar linear character of most policy programmes and paradigms.

"I am working in a factory . . ."

The social work practitioner[1] quoted at the start of this chapter worked in a local authority child care team and, with those words, was opening an exploration of her experience of the impact on her organization of "audit culture" and the regime of inspection that accompanies the *Every Child Matters* policy stream (DfES, 2003). She continued:

> We produce initial and core assessments in our factory. Our management counts the assessments completed on a weekly basis and informs the workers of the results in teams meetings and by emails. The workers don't seem to care about these numbers but they preoccupy the management.
>
> There have been many changes in our factory in the past five years, due to demands from above and competition from other factories. The management has been replaced, the teams were reconstructed, the machinery (workers, forms, IT systems) also saw great changes.
>
> I am quite confused about who is my master and who do I need to serve. Is it the customer or is it the government, and do they have conflicting interests? I am thinking of running away from this factory, to look for another job . . . in another factory.

Later she writes of how:

> The management measures (in percentages) the reports of initial and core assessments completed on time, and compares these to other teams. When the team manager reports these statistics in team meetings, I can recognize how my body becomes tense and my heart rate increases, and I get very angry. When we do not meet in team meetings, we often receive emails about the statistics, and I have the same bodily reaction. I have voiced my resentment to this ritual, but it was ignored by managers and other colleagues.

Speaking of her organization, she says:

> In order to adjust practice to inspection standards our organization has become:
>
> Obsessive about records
>
> Obsessive about statistics
>
> Manipulative of the statistics.

Then once again speaking of herself, but now from a more theorized perspective:

> Throughout the policy process seminar [on the post-qualifying course on which she was a student] I found I held negative attitudes towards the government and the organization, their policies and procedures. I now realize that I was caught up in a dynamic process involving the mirroring of defences and anxieties (on the part of) government, the organization, and practitioners.

She describes this dynamic process as a "triangle of tension" in which there is a kind of game of "passing the painful parcel". Government concerns to generate social improvement within self-imposed limited budgets and short time scales dovetail with lack of trust in professionals and target cultures that project anxiety and responsibility downwards onto provider organizations, which, fearful about their own "performance" and survival, in turn project these anxieties into staff. The central anxiety for all parties is something like: "We will fail, be seen to have failed, and then we will be blamed and annihilated"; the dominant defence is to project responsibility and the associated anxiety about failure, blame, and survival downwards, demand that performance be measurable and measured in order to avoid conditions that produce failure, but then punish any failures to meet performance standards. The writer quotes Michael Power's (1994) observation that "Audit creates the pathologies for which it is the prescribed treatment".

As an illustration of how to take emotional experience as the point of departure for policy analysis, this is as good as any. Equally, it is not a template. But various features of her account open the door to an appreciation of some of the components that constitute our emerging model of psycho-social policy analysis. I examine some of these in turn.

Emotions: local intelligence, global significance

First, specific social and political relationships are revealed to be inscribed within particular emotional experiences. The meaning of specific feelings and emotional conflicts, in the context of organizational role performance, are illuminated and rendered legible in the light of a theoretically informed reflective policy analysis. At the same time, the immediate, visceral character of lived emotional experience—physical tension, increased heart rate, anger—is not reductively eliminated, pathologized, or explained away. Rather, it becomes available as a vital source of "intelligence", a resource that can inform understanding of the organizational and policy "life world". This viewpoint extends somewhat the work of David Armstrong (2004) on "Emotions in Organizations: Disturbance or Intelligence?" to include the policy domain, itself a key determinant of public sector organizational processes and cultures. Of organizational life, Armstrong says:

> No organization stands alone, insulated from its context, any more than each of us, as individuals, stands alone. While that context is relatively stable or predictable, it may be taken as given, something to which an organization needs continually to adapt, but without having fundamentally to question either what it does or how it does it.
>
> However, few organizations at present, either those we are members of or those we work with, inhabit such a context. Correspondingly our experience in and of organizations now is probably being shaped by challenges from without as much as, if not more than, anxieties from within. Since these challenges are registered emotionally, we suggest that they have to do not only with questions of viability, whether or not the organization will survive, but equally with the *cost* of viability, what will and what must be risked in the cause of survival. [Armstrong, 2004, p. 24, emphasis in original]

At the conclusion of this piece, Armstrong says:

> No emotional experience in organizational life is a suitable case for treatment. It is rather a resource for thinking, for releasing intelligence. [p. 27]

A consistent "finding" of the method of policy analysis outlined in this chapter is that by approaching the emotional experience of policy actors not as a "symptom" of either individual psychological functioning, or even exclusively of organizational life, but, rather, as a registration of the complexities, contradictions, anxieties, and defences inherent within policy processes, one can move outwards from "subjective experience" to embrace analysis of the global forces now acting on the inherently "unstable" national policy environment we all inhabit. In this way, moment-by-moment emotional particularities—the very fabric and texture of everyday lived experience—can be located as meaningful registrations of the nature of complex social and political processes.

Conflict—critique or resistance?

The practitioner finds herself professionally and emotionally conflicted in the face of the policy-driven organizational and professional transformations she experiences and records. There is a suggestion of wanting to challenge and resist, or at least negotiate a different kind of accommodation to these changes, and she notes the emergence of a split between the concerns of managers and of front-line staff like herself. But her attempts to voice her frustration lead nowhere.

Audit and inspection regimes are an integral part of the "new public sector", its enactment through the doctrines of "new public management", and are structurally tied to the wider reconstruction of the economics, politics, and culture of public policy within emerging "market states" (Cooper, 2008c; Wilson, Ruch, Lymbery, & Cooper, 2008). From the perspective of everyday lived experience, these are genuinely transformative processes, but not ones in relation to which citizens have really been offered choice, consultation, or even much public debate.

One can interpret or find meaning in the practitioner's registration of her conflicted experience in several possible ways. First, it seems to mark how, in the absence of strong intermediate collectives capable of engaging with the political process, controversial processes of social change with powerful impacts upon deprived populations and the public services with whom they relate may no longer be an object of public contestation. What might once have registered and been available at the level of social conflict becomes, instead, inscribed as part of subjective experience.

Second, the possibility of critique, let alone of action, seems to be muted or suppressed in this individual's experience. She reports feeling "negative" towards her organization and towards government, with the implication that this was experienced as a "feeling without form", until she could avail herself of a *theory* that made sense of her emotional experience. Perhaps this goes to the heart of questions about epistemology and psycho-social ontology implied by this model of policy analysis. Psycho-social *experience* is taken to *precede* articulated *knowledge* of our conditions of existence, as much as to follow from such knowledge or discursive location. This is a realist position, but not a simple one. Real-world social processes may be registered as emotional experience, but they stand in need of concepts or appropriate categories of thought if they are to become "thinkable" and hence available as a basis for critique or, indeed, genuine *consent*.

So, third, the sense for this individual of being an "object" and not a "subject" of policy becomes associated with a tendency to resist policy-led change rather than engage with it. Elsewhere she makes clear that she does not wholly oppose the aspirations of modern inspection and audit regimes, and for any of us some policy initiatives will be broadly welcome, some not, while to many we will have mixed responses. But as "active citizens" we respond to social change not just as an expression of "values" we hold or oppose, or as instruments guiding us towards ends, but as emotionally meaningful interventions that impact upon our developed sense of what it is to be part of a "flourishing social order". Denied the opportunity or a public language with which to engage with change on the basis of the fullness of our responses, we may resist changes we would otherwise welcome, comply resentfully with those we would question or resist, or any perverse combination of these. This is surely bad news for policymakers. The more cynical conclusion to be drawn from this analysis is that by enabling fuller engagement and participation in policy processes, policymakers are more likely to "get what they want" whether people ultimately agree with the change process in question or not; more hopefully, a truly flourishing society may be one in which there is more, not less, open social conflict, debate, and contestation—although policy-led change may be rather harder to "deliver on time" under such circumstances.

Resistance to policy change receives remarkably little attention in the literature. Yet, how and why people resist is of instrumental significance and interest to policymakers, as well as to our critical engagement with policy processes. The naturalistic psycho-social study of policy actors as they negotiate unfolding real-world policy conditions would be a significant development in policy studies.

Non-linearity

Until very recently, the notion of policy implementation as a process of "muddling through" is the nearest that mainstream analysts have come to questioning the "linearity" of policy processes. From a rational linear perspective, policy failures are explained in terms of the internal logic of implementation itself, rather than the interaction between implementation and the wider social system in which implementation occurs. Traditional policy analysis still relies upon a machine metaphor to "diagnose" social ills, and "treat" them to effect a "cure"; but societies are not machines, and they are better conceptualized as complex adaptive systems, or social ecologies, in which the relationship between causes and effects are non-linear and never fully predictable. Policy processes are systemic interventions, which *inevitably* generate unanticipated and unpredictable consequences that undermine or distort the effort to achieve pre-established goals. Recognizing these realities, successful policy implementation is likely to depend on learning from experience and on reflexive adaptation of processes in response to emerging evidence of the holistic impact of interventions in a complex social totality.

This concept of policy processes has been elaborated by Jake Chapman in a publication aptly titled *System Failure: Why Governments Must Learn to Think Differently* (2004). Resistance to change is as much a "natural" feature of complex human systems as receptivity or compliance, and it is essentially emotionally rooted, but to embrace resistance (or "make an ally of it", in psychoanalytic parlance) rather than attempt to overrule it requires ceding the illusion of absolute control over change processes. The necessity for authentic collaboration enters the picture and thus, also, a negotiative, participatory model of social relations to replace the tendency towards "command and control" that remains the default mode of conventional policymaking.

Death and the mandarin: social fantasy and the roots of policy

Realist social policy analysis locates policy as an aspect of the social totality *as it is*, not as policy wishes it to be (even if the nature of what "is" continues to be contested, as it surely will be). A systemic stance towards policy enables us to take up a meta-perspective on our own policy-related experience and activity and to situate policy processes in real-world understanding. Once this shift of perspective is achieved, policy processes are disclosed as shaped and impelled by many forces beyond those recognized by the traditional policy paradigm itself; equally they are revealed to contribute to the emerging character of social relations not apparently primarily driven by policy imperatives.

The practitioner quoted above sees inspection and audit regimes as manifestations of governmental and social anxiety and as processes that shape and intersect with the inherent anxieties of the organizational and professional task of child care social work. The relationship between anxiety and organizational structure, culture and functioning has been fruitfully developed within psychoanalytic practice and theory (Menzies, 1959; Obholzer & Zagier Roberts, 1994), but as with Armstrong's analysis of emotion in organizations (2004), this can readily be extended to embrace wider social formations.

When, for example, we stand back from the sense of political urgency that follows a major public disaster or tragedy, and from the rapid policy prescriptions that normally ensue, it is possible to discern the complex interplay of rationality and irrationality, reason and emotion, that structures them. Quality assurance regimes, risk-management protocols, public inquiries, and standards audits are all, on the face of it, eminently sensible efforts to reduce risk and prevent avoidable future harm. However, a steady focus on what lies "under the surface" of these responses can disclose a more complex picture in which deep anxieties about responsibility for damage and death are being "rationally managed" rather than faced and tolerated or worked through socially (see also chapters 6 and 7 of this book). "Risk society" is surely a product of our emotional encounter with new kinds of social "dangers", but the concept of, for example, "low-probability–high-consequence" risks and their disproportionate impact on *universal* policy responses, despite the small chance of their occurrence, alerts us to the difficulty at the level of the "social unconscious" of knowing how to respond rationally to events—and importantly the *fear* of events—that are almost literally unthinkable. If a fear is unthinkable, then it cannot be symbolized within ordinary discourse, or its symbolization may be so imbued with elements of fantasy and anxiety that the "rational" is massively impregnated by currents of "irrationality".

Rational instrumental policy processes generated under such conditions—in the wake of nuclear accident, sadistic child murder, insulin murders by health care staff, organized sexual abuse of children, terrorist attacks, and so on—are inscribed with the emotional charge and dangerousness of their origins. Emotional responses to tragic and disturbing events may be individually and socially "legible" but equally they may not, evoking our most primitive anxieties and panicky, inchoate social impulses to defend ourselves. In our work on these matters, we have found that death and the fear of death makes itself known as a frequent and frequently unacknowledged source of policy anxiety. In a striking observation, Obholzer (1994) characterized the NHS as a "save us all from death" service. But in the context of how prevalent is death as a shaping experience in policy processes, consider Bauman's thoughts on the question:

> And there are more than enough reasons for the consciousness of mortality to be traumatic. First and foremost, thinking about death defies thought itself . . . reason's power is to be a guide to good choice, but death is not a matter of choice. Death is a scandal, the ultimate humiliation of reason. [Bauman, 1992, pp. 14–15]

The structuring role of social fantasy in policymaking has been explored by Evans (2003) with respect to sexual offenders; Cooper and Lousada (2005) in relation to audit and governance regimes, child abuse, and child death; Taylor (2007) in his exploration of NHS clinical governance regimes; and Cooper (2008a) with respect to the public disclosure of murders within health care systems. Showalter (1997) surveys a range of moral panics and phantom epidemics in her wide-ranging study *Hystories*. If policy programmes are taken to be just a part of life and not an omnipotent solution to all life's ills and anxieties, then they might succeed more often when their own limits are acknowledged more often and more readily. Psychoanalytically we might call this "depressive-position" policymaking; better, perhaps, to think of it as common-sense policymaking.

The critical imagination

Without access to this domain of emotional experience, it is hard to imagine how the satirical narrative of "factory life" with which the writer opens her account could have been written. We sometimes speak of satire as "biting", and this reflects the anger, and the emotional as well as intellectual critique, that constitutes this literary mode of engagement with experience. If emotional responses can be a form of "information" about our psycho-social conditions of existence, then what of imagination?

Social facts and methodologically sound analyses of quantitative data sets will always be important in good policy analysis—we cannot rationally propose to commit public resources to projects solely on the basis of emotional responses or leaps of social imagination, not least because these can just as easily serve distorting and destructive ends as progressive and creative ones if they are uncoupled from rational inquiry. The organized racist imagination, for example, is nourished by specific "material conditions" of social life such as economic deprivation but misreads, or selectively articulates, the nature of the facts as well as the explanation of these facts. But the strength of a "grounded" imaginative register of engagement with policy processes and political life is to heal the split between the scientistic and the speculative, the so-called subjective and objective registers of analysis. The psychoanalyst D. W. Winnicott (1971a) observed that the intermediate realm between our inner world of personal experience and the outer world of external reality is "the place where we live". As creatures who daily inhabit, but also negotiate and influence, a world shaped by policy processes, the same intermediate area of "potential experience" must be one point of departure for analysis and engagement with policy.

Conclusion

In an era of evidence-based practice and policymaking that privileges measurable data suitable for the requirements of audit, rational evaluation, and transparency, literary evidence will struggle to achieve impact. Historically, however, literature has made a considerable contribution to social reform. The novels of Charles Dickens are a well-documented instance, and today a minor tradition of critical documentary and feature-film-making survives to continue this tradition. Arguably emotionality, passion, and social criticism find their most articulate meeting point in such work. The exclusion of both from mainstream policy analysis discloses something important about the political times in which we live. Psycho-social work on emotion and public policy aspires to reclaim something of the wholeness of lived experience for the political process; however, this means "listening" to our experience in new and perhaps unfamiliar ways and seeking means by which others can be persuaded to listen differently in turn.

Note

1. This presentation was made in the context of the practitioner's work on a module entitled "The Policy Process", which is part of the University of East London/Tavistock Centre MA/Professional Doctorate in Advanced Social Work. She did not wish to be named or her organization identified, although she was happy to be cited in this chapter. This decision directly reflects themes discussed above concerning the suppression of critical debate about policy processes in a contemporary "survivalist" policy culture, as well as the dissolution of institutions that support the voices and interests of groups in civil society impacted by everyday political and policy processes. I am grateful to this colleague for agreeing that her work could be quoted in this chapter.

PART IV

RESEARCH

CHAPTER TWELVE

Hearing the grass grow: emotional and epistemological challenges of practice-near research

> "In this job you have to talk to people about things that really no one should ever be made to talk about."
>
> Child protection social worker

Twenty-two corpses

I am a fan, or in truth I should say an addict, of the American TV series *The Wire*. Set in the city of Baltimore, the five seasons of *The Wire* explore the complex inter-relationships between the police department, the drug dealers, suppliers, and addicts of the streets and corners—many of whom are children—and the politicians and the media. Part of what engrosses me about *The Wire* is that it is like watching ethnography on TV, and if a really good TV series were ever made about social work I think it would necessarily have some of the characteristics of *The Wire*. Terrible things happen in the course of the narrative that unfolds. Near the end of Season 4, twenty-two decomposing bodies are discovered by police in separate locations in derelict houses in the city. These are the corpses of various people executed by Marlo, the dominant West Side drug dealer and his hit-man and hit-woman, because they became inconvenient—they snitched, they were rivals, and so on.

The promotional statement on the Season 5 DVD box begins by saying: "In a city that can no longer even recognize its problems, much less begin to solve them, police detectives attempt to bring in one last worthy case against a violent crew of narcotics traffickers" (HBO, 2008). This idea—of a city that can no longer recognize its problems—intrigued me. A few years ago I wrote a book with a colleague about the changing nature of the welfare state project in Britain, in which we proposed that one of the functions of an organized welfare state was to enable society to recognize, tolerate the knowledge of, and act upon its own problems (Cooper & Lousada, 2005). In one chapter (but see also chapter 8 of the present book), I used the example of the Cleveland sexual abuse crisis of the late 1980s to explore how our social and professional capacity to tolerate new "dangerous knowledge" about ourselves and the society we inhabit cannot be taken for granted. The outcome of that crisis was broadly that we accepted the much greater prevalence of sexual abuse in our midst. But at the time it was a tremendous contest with an uncertain resolution. Powerful groupings fought hard in the public domain to deny that there was any validity to what was being uncovered. At the time, many of us did not know what to believe or think. This was partly because we did not have a proper conceptual apparatus at either a personal or a social level with which to think the difficult thoughts about the unwelcome realities that were emerging for the public into the light of day.

Just down the street

In 2008 and 2009, I think something of the same climate was evident in the wake of the trial of Baby P's killers, their sentencing, and the eventual disclosure of their identities. The atmosphere during the weeks when this tragic case was at the forefront of media and political attention in Britain felt very different from that which surrounded the last big "child abuse scandal" in Britain—the death of Victoria Climbié and the Public Inquiry that ensued. At the height of the "Baby P" crisis, the public domain felt unusually volatile, as though there was a chance that government might do something truly panic-stricken and damaging to the social work profession, or that the vigilante climate might result in the murder or suicide of one of the social work staff involved, although by the end of the most acute period there was also a sense of a better realization in government and in the public sphere of what the realities of child protection work entail.

At the height of this period of anxiety, I wrote an article in a national newspaper (Cooper, 2008b) saying that some people who abuse and torture children *need* to carry on doing this. They are expelling something intolerable, dangerous, and murderous in themselves into someone else and might be severely destabilized in themselves if stopped. They also usually know what they are doing, and that it is a dreadful crime. For them, the stakes could not be higher in relation to those people—social workers—charged with recognizing and naming what is happening.

When social work is accused of "failing", I tend to think that the charge is really that we have failed at a certain point to shield the general public from *awareness* of those very realities that we do succeed, most of the time, in protecting people from having to contemplate. And maybe a bigger proportion of the public understand this than we imagine is the case. As I said previously, during the week when the Baby P crisis was at its height, the most intelligent conversation I felt I had was with a London cab driver who said, "I can't read about that case in the papers—it's too distressing . . . I couldn't do that job, I wouldn't be able to sleep at night." He laughed a little nervously and looked at me in the mirror, and said, "I suppose I wouldn't have been a very good social worker." This is one thing social workers do at a societal level—help people sleep at night, not because we are defending the realm against communists, terrorists, or insurgents, but because we are protecting people from the emotional impact of knowing about the torture of babies that may be happening just down the street.

Ugly facts

Research is about generating "new knowledge", but in my view it is also about enlarging the scope of our self-knowledge in the personal, professional, and societal domains. We need sound methodologies for conducting research of any kind, but actually we can only hope to generate new knowledge insofar as we are emotionally and ideologically open to the possibility of discovering something new, including things we really did not want to know. If we are blind to or defended against this possibility, then the best methodologies may not help us much, although we should recognize that the formal properties of many research methodologies exist precisely in order to ensure systematic open-mindedness. Charles Darwin apparently referred to the necessity of first collecting the "ugly facts" if we are to hope to build a beautiful theory. But we know from the work of Kuhn (1975) and others on paradigm shifts that even the collection of "ugly" or inconvenient facts may not disturb a settled world view, until that world view is ready to be disturbed or until someone proposes an alternative theory that embraces everything explained by the old one, as well as the inconvenient facts it couldn't account for. This is so much more the case in psycho-social research and social life than it is in the material or life sciences, because the world we are investigating is *our* world—a construct of meanings, affects, relationships, and so on that can never be fully independent of the researcher, or the knowing subject, with his or her theoretical, personal, and ideological commitments.

This view of research in social work, and I will shortly come to the question of "practice-near" research, sets it decisively apart from other views of research which try to keep faith with something I will call "proper science" for short—the proponents of the possibility of "objective knowledge" to be acquired through "proper" scientific method. I think that practice-near social work research is, or should be, part of a total world view of sufficient power and legitimacy to rival that which the "proper scientists" have the privilege and security of occupying. We are some way from achieving this in relation to practice-near research, if it is even a goal to which we would aspire—since it may be that many proponents of qualitative social research think the idea of a single, stable, secure, and settled epistemological world view with respect to psycho-social worlds is a rather dangerous illusion.

So what does practice-near research involve? What does it give us? What is its implied world view, if any? My thoughts about this are based partly on the kinds of things I believe it should be and should deliver, but also on the kinds of things it *is* delivering in my experience—though in truth this is mostly not based on my first-hand experience but on that of doctoral students whom I have been privileged to work with over the years. "Practice" is about people, relationships, and organizations and social systems such as teams and networks made up of people and relationships. If we want to ask what it might mean to get "near" to practice, then we might rephrase the question as "What happens when we get *close*, emotionally or physically, to people?" Here are a few of the possible answers I can think of, which I will try to illustrate with examples from recent research. Each item is, in fact, intertwined with all the others:

1. The smell of the real: practice-near research will bring us close to people in a visceral, bodily, and therefore live emotional way. This can be exciting, or perturbing, or both, but, whatever, it is likely to be hard to stay "objective" or "dispassionate" in research endeavours of this kind. Practice-near research will be passionate research about passions, in which the boundaries of the researcher's self

are likely to become fluid and uncertain. Consequently, we need methodologies that can help us with the intensity and epistemological uncertainties that arise from such research encounters.

2. Losing our minds: the closer we come to other people, the greater the likelihood that we will become psychically mixed up with them. This could be because we fall in love with them, because we hate or despise them with inexplicable intensity, or we swing between the two, or any of a thousand other ways we have of entangling ourselves one with another. We all need other people to project into, and so of course others are doing this with us, and often we accept these projections without realizing that they are not "us". We lose parts of ourselves in others and find ourselves inhabited by the lost parts of others. You can deny that all this is so, and that is your perfect right. But if you accept it, or something like it, then you will need a theoretical account of how such processes operate in order successfully to manage the research act and to extricate yourself from potential confusion.
3. The inevitability of personal change: the psychological intensity of these kinds of encounters changes us, whether we wish for this or not. Thus, I have come to the conclusion that a test of whether something really is "practice-near" research might be whether or not the researcher felt themselves to be changed as a person in the course of the work.
4. The discovery of "complex particulars": if you are close enough to your research subject for all the above to be happening, then you will not be engaged with large populations of research subjects. But just because you are studying specific cases or a small range of "particulars", this does not mean the research has no wider or even universal significance. The closer one comes to a single case, the more its uniqueness and particularity demands to be understood, but, equally, the more its value for the illumination of all other cases with which there is a family resemblance becomes evident. This view of matters poses, in my view, a fundamental challenge to the continuing dominance of a positivist world view.

In the following pages, I present some quite lengthy extracts from the work of a number of researchers. By and large, I do not comment on these. The message in relation to the theme each of them illustrates should be self-evident, but also I hope that readers will allow the material to stimulate their own associations, anxieties, and thoughts and that some time is taken to then reflect on these responses.

(1) The smell of the real

When we come close to people, we become directly aware of their bodies, and they of ours—we smell them, even if we aren't touching them. We may like what we smell and be attracted to them, or we may be repulsed by their bad breath or body odour. Probably we find it difficult to be emotionally neutral about being so near to someone. But if, let's say, we encounter an unpleasant smell, we may reflect that it is difficult for people to smell themselves. If people were aware of their powerful bad breath, for example, they would presumably take steps to prevent it more often than they seem to; however, such reflections may mean we start to wonder anxiously about our own body odours—or, perturbed by these thoughts, we may try *not* to think them. This, of course, is the kind of territory that Isabel Menzies Lyth was disclosing to us in her classic 1959 paper "A Case Study in the Functioning of Social Systems as a Defence against Anxiety" (Menzies, 1959) in which she theorized about the impact on hospital organizational life of the daily experience of nurses in close emotional and physical contact with patients.

In her study of the dynamics and processes that underlie critical incidents in high-security settings such as special hospitals, Jude Deacon (2010) recorded and analysed a variety of long-term consultations and supervisory processes with workers who are subject to the kinds of emotional and organizational pressures likely to be encountered on a daily basis by staff working in such settings with very disturbed and dangerous people. As with many of the public inquiries into health and welfare "failures" and critical incidents, the prominent ones from high-security settings signally fail to really show us *how* the "failure" occurred or the process by which a breakdown in professional functioning developed. Deacon's research aims to fill this gap in understanding, working from the assumption that the processes that explain such incidents are more likely everyday ones rather being than exceptional or aberrant.

Here Deacon presents data from a subject in the institution where she worked at the time, to whom at the outset she was offering clinical supervision, but for whom she later had also line-management responsibility.

Ms A from 23/05/05:

Ms A said that she had "an issue" she would like to raise with me about a member of the team. She named one of the men and said that she thought he "might have a problem with alcohol". He had been noted by various members of the team, clearly for some time, to be smelling of alcohol. She said "I've thought about saying to him—you regularly smell of alcohol but I thought it seemed confrontational. And yet, role-playing saying it to you just then, I can see that it's not confrontational."

She confirmed that he had had a lot of sickness absence and also had appalling timekeeping. In the past, before she was acting-up, "we used to joke about it all the time—'where's Z?'" He would not turn in for work and not contact the department. She knew that he was living in London and would always get held up in traffic—arrive at lunchtime. She used to think "why doesn't he just leave earlier?" She also knows that he works as a musician at nights. There have been occasions when he has come to work smelling of alcohol and has clearly not been to bed. The timekeeping has improved somewhat since he got a room in the nurses' hostel on site. But there are still issues. One of the other men had recently refused to share an office with him "because he always stinks". Although the colleague had not specified alcohol, she knew that was what he meant.

Ms A from 22/06/05:

... Ms A was also proposing to the team that she be enabled to contact tutors to confirm their attendance when they attended external courses for Continuing Professional Development. One team member (Z) had claimed regular time off in lieu for attendance at a course. However, a colleague, on the same course, had alerted Ms A to the fact that Z's attendance had been poor. This person had passed with flying colours but Z had been granted a year's extension on his final assignment ...

... She spoke again of Z's absences, saying that it was funny that the rest of the team spoke so little to her about these absences now. In the past, before she was acting-head of the dept, the subject of Z's absences was "a standing joke"—they were always joking about the fact that Z "was never there—'where's Z? Don't know!'" She recalled a time, when he had only recently joined the team, and he was found asleep in a therapy room. Her predecessor had dealt with it ...

A small section of the researcher's analysis of this data reads as follows:

> It is clear from her descriptions that over a substantial period of time the team had grown accustomed to colluding with Z's behaviour. In a collective denial of the seriousness and potential consequences of such behaviour, they *"used to joke about it all the time"*.

> Indeed it had become *"a standing joke"* that they are collectively holding as a secret: a dangerous secret. The risk and ethical implications of the member of staff smelling of alcohol and indeed quite possibly being intoxicated or otherwise incapable of effective work were completely absent from the material as were any references to the clear breaches of Trust policies or the code of conduct required by the Health Professions Council with whom therapists maintain professional registration. Similarly, she does not acknowledge the aggression and denial of reality implicit in his behaviour. It would seem that Z's potential risk is not taken seriously. In response I felt it necessary to introduce this framework of boundaries into the sessions, to clarify her role in this regard and to be prescriptive with her as to what actions she should take in order to avoid the service being further compromised by this man both in the short and long terms. [Deacon, 2010, p. 111]

(2) Losing our minds

In research that is truly "practice-near", we risk losing a clear sense of where the boundary lies between ourselves and other people. We also see this in our observations of research subjects—for example, that they may often appear to be ensnared in repetitive, destructive dynamics with one another in which its clear that individuals are actually parts of a psychic or psycho-social system, or they may be lost in some kind of mutual idealization in which each is needed by the other to sustain the illusion of admiration—but we too will experience it in our relationship as researchers to our research subjects. An apparently stray, unbidden, but powerful thought or memory suddenly enters our awareness, related to what we are observing or discussing in an interview, but also clearly *our* thought. Or is it so clear? Why, at that precise moment, that particular thought? Here we are in the territory explored by the psychoanalyst Thomas Ogden in his work on the nature, experience, and meaning of the therapist's "reverie" in clinical sessions (Ogden, 1999). Ultimately he evokes an idea of the patient–analyst pair creating a kind of "psychic field", both unconscious and conscious, between them. Thus, particular "reveries" do have a meaning that extends beyond the individual and can, in Ogden's view, be used to access aspects of unconscious experience in the patient.

In her study of three front-line social work teams, Judy Foster (2009) makes use of this kind of recording and interpretation of her own emotional experience; but she also cites a cautionary passage from Christopher Bollas (1987) about the status of "countertransference experiences":

> Counter-transference readiness creates an internal space which allows for a more complete and articulate expression of the patient's transference speech than if I were to close down this internal space and replace it with some ideal notion of absolute mental neutrality or scientific detachment. . . . This inevitable, ever-present, and necessary uncertainty about why we feel as we do gives to our private ongoing consideration of the counter-transference a certain humility and responsibility. [Foster, 2009, pp. 202–203]

In Foster's presentation and discussion of her lengthy series of observations and interviews with a hospital social work team, there are the following passages:

> *Desolation and despair*
>
> "There was one old lady like a little sparrow who had pushed her chair out so as to catch people as they walked by the end of her bed, repeating "Are you the Doctor? I want to go home" in the most distressing way. Her cotton robe was hanging open at the chest and I felt very confused as to whether to stop and straighten it for her. But what would I do when she clung to me? And would that make it worse? I walked on to the meeting room, disturbed by the scene and my feelings" (Visit 5H).
>
> On the following day I returned with Gail (one of the social workers) to a ward with twenty-eight beds for older people who had suffered strokes. I was assailed by the sense of desolation and despair. The meeting did nothing to alleviate this since only the consultant and the ward doctor spoke. The other nine participants sat silently for two hours. There was no attempt to develop a rapport between staff or to use the meeting to explore problems and dilemmas. The oppressive attitude of the consultant seemed to mirror the repression of any life and individuality in the patients. Perhaps signs of life would lead to more despair by patients, which staff were not equipped to tolerate. Perhaps the staff's confusion on the best way forward would be the same as mine? I spent the time preoccupied, worried that my father-in-law was in a similar ward. My notes were as monosyllabic and lifeless as the meeting.
>
> *A personal interlude*
>
> My personal situation was entwined with the observation and influenced my perceptions of it. My elderly parents-in-law were reaching the end

> of their long lives. They lived in their own home with some daily help for my father-in-law. When he could no longer climb the stairs, he was admitted to the local hospital for assessment. After the second Multi-Disciplinary Team meeting referred to above, I visited him the next day. We had a remarkable talk. This consoled us when he died suddenly the following morning. I stopped my observation for two weeks for the funeral and returned for the month of February, conscious of another break in relation to the team. In my last week, my mother-in-law was living alone for the first time in her life, with the prospect of all her children being out of contact for the following week. We were all pre-occupied and anxious as to how we could help her "hold it together."

(3) The inevitability of personal change

Practice-near research changes the researcher and may change or transform research subjects. Insofar as the research act is itself an interpretive one, in which the "truth" of the data is in part dependent on the interpretive framework of the researcher, there can even be a meaningful sense in which "reality itself" is transformed in the process of the research; however, for this to happen, the researcher herself may (no, will) have to undergo a parallel transformation.

In her paper "Projective Processes on the Front Line" Sylvia Smith (2007), a very experienced black practitioner and manager, describes a research consultation interview, her subsequent research journal reflections on this interview, and then a process in which she suddenly "saw the data differently". She likens this to what the psychoanalyst Wilfred Bion called a shift in "vertex".

The data episode in question is dense, but I will do my best to encapsulate it. It concerns an account given in a research consultation session by two social work managers of a children's centre, a sequence of events involving (a) a black male service user who was the father of (b) a baby girl with whom he has "contact sessions" at the centre where the research was undertaken. During Contact Session 1, (c) a white social worker and (d) a white deputy project manager are reported to have found the service user angry and intimidating, and as a result his contact is terminated. His contact is later reinstated by (e) the black project manager and (f) a new black deputy project manager.

At a second contact session, a centre worker (g) challenged the service user because he persistently removed the bottle from his daughter's mouth as she was feeding; during this contact session the baby's black Children's Guardian (h) arrives (seemingly unexpectedly) and at more or less the same time the black deputy project manager (f) also entered the room. Later the Guardian reportedly commented to the deputy manager that *"had she been alone in the room with the service user, he would have probably attacked her"* (Smith, 2007, p. 211).

Following Contact Session 1, the deputy manager had (i) met the service user who seems to have acknowledged that he had been "intimidating" to centre staff; however, (ii) the deputy manager had suggested to him that he had not been intimidating or aggressive but merely disputed the arrangements in some way, and (iii) had subsequently talked to the white centre worker who had agreed that "with hindsight the service user had not in fact been hostile or aggressive, but that perhaps with hindsight the worker's anxiety and hysteria about what could potentially have happened had been fuelled by the service user's non-responsiveness to centre staff on that day . . ." (Smith, 2007, p. 210).

In her commentary, Smith describes how in the research consultation

> As a black person hearing this account from another black person, I strongly identified with all the thoughts and feelings of the service user about being misunderstood as a race of people by white professionals. As the Deputy Manager shared this account there was a shared "understanding" among the three of us as black people, in terms of the ease with which we are often perceived as "aggressive and intimidating". [2007, p. 211]

However, as she reviews her written data record, Smith begins to see the "interpretation" of events implied in the above commentary in a different light. She wonders whether it might not be quite plausible that the service user became angry; she wonders whether the centre worker might have found it difficult to challenge the deputy manager's interpretation of events at Contact Session 1 "for fear of being accused of racism"; and she suggests that in Contact Session 2 the Guardian "could clearly see the danger, but we (deputy manager, project manager and I) were more preoccupied with the Guardian's remarks and how misunderstood this service user was and how unjustly he had been perceived" (2007, p. 211).

But this "shift of perspective" is not a consequence just of "rational reflection", or systematic "reanalysis" of the data. Something else intervenes, and Smith says:

> I recalled an incident which took place some time ago when I was a team manager . . . During a very busy day I had joined a member of staff to support her with a very angry client and his partner in an

> interview room. They were a black couple. The service user was a black man who had become very verbally abusive in the meeting and seemed to channel most of his anger towards me. I remained quite calm as he shouted and "ranted" on for several minutes . . . I later met with my line manager to debrief about what had taken place. She immediately felt the danger in the incident . . . It was only during this discussion with my line manager that it began to dawn on me the potential danger this incident presented. [2007, pp. 212–213]

This piece of analysis and reflection captures in a complex fashion several inter-related aspects of the research process. First, the data decisively does *not* speak for itself: when the researcher is in identification with her research subjects and their view of the world, reality is one thing; when she questions her identifications, then the whole pattern of interpretation shifts and in some respects inverts. All the evidence for this revised interpretation was available first time round, but some of the facts were, let's say, "inconvenient"; however, the shift of perspective seems to be enabled or supported by an internal process in the researcher, a kind of "reverie", in fact, that comes to her aid in the form of a memory of another shift in perspective involving questions of race, aggression, and dangerousness. Perhaps it is significant that the recollected incident involves a seemingly trusted black manager, but whatever the case this figure is the one the researcher now identifies with, and who represents the capacity for her to "observe her own research ego" and take up a "third position" with respect to the data.

Analysis like this brings me closer to an understanding of the social world in which the fluid and recursive nature of time and experience is similar to that captured so eloquently in T. S. Eliot's *Four Quartets* (1962). This is a view of the nature of reality far from compatible with "proper science" and its methods and assumptions about linear causality. The only question for me is, how seriously do we take this more mysterious conception of social reality? And do we have the courage to really fight for its legitimacy in our professional dealings?

Maybe this is also the right point to note something that has been implicit throughout most of what I have said so far: emotional experience and epistemology seem to me to be inextricably entangled in this kind of research, a topic that is more fully explored in chapter 15. I think the conventional view about sound research methodology is that it protects the research(er) from the distorting influence of his or her subjectivity and emotional responses; good practice-near research seems to me to *depend* on subjectivity and emotional engagement with the object of research. What, then, can safeguard us against the prejudices and distortions of the researcher's passions? I think it can only be the kind of mental and emotional flexibility that Sylvia Smith's example illustrates, and which convinces us because of the depth of analysis it supports.

Certain kinds of research—notably, action research—set out to effect change in the subjects being researched. But there is a good deal of evidence that the kind of work I have been presenting may create change in ways that cannot be planned, anticipated, or contracted for.

Another of Jude Deacon's (2010) research subjects was a police child protection officer, who volunteered to engage in a series of consultative interviews about his work. The hope was that this might provide depth insight into the kinds of psychological pressures exerted by suspects with a great deal to lose on someone carrying authority and responsibility for getting at the truth of his actions. And so it proved, I think, but over the months we realized that another process was at work, in which the meaning of the consultations for the subject seemed to involve a gradual awareness or acceptance that he found this work intolerable.

> *DC B from 26/07/05:*
>
> He said that it had been a "really strange" few weeks. He thought that things had "been getting on top" of him—then he had been ill for 2 weeks—he had been to a barbeque and got food poisoning followed by an infection—and then he had had a week's pre-booked leave. He spoke of the nature of our work, saying that he felt "relatively comfortable" talking to sex offenders but that there were other aspects of the work that were more difficult. One of his colleagues had told him about a job she was working on. It was a case of neglect of a young baby. The child had been so badly neglected that it had resorted to eating its own faeces. DC B had found this very difficult to deal with. Again he said that things seemed to have got on top of him a little . . .
>
> *DC B from 06/12/05:*
>
> He had been speaking to a female colleague in their office when something she said (either he didn't tell me or, as I write this up, I cannot recall what it was that she said) made him "blub", tears streaming down his face. "You bitch", he said to her. I asked him where that had come from ("you bitch")—was it not entirely understandable that he would be moved by such a perverse crime? He said that he thought it might have been because it was in front of all their team. He then moved very swiftly on saying "and then I got a job that really did make me cry" . . .

> . . . DC B had then gone home. He was sitting with his young son, who, he said, is "not usually a very demonstrative child". His son had suddenly flung his arms around him, and DC B had found himself moved to tears. He had excused himself from his son saying he would go and get him a drink. He then went outside until he could compose himself. He said that he didn't want to have to explain to his son why he was crying.
>
> *DC B from 06/12/05:*
>
> DC B then said he felt he'd had enough and couldn't take any more. He laughed as he said it but said that he thought if he "had to hear one more thing about someone's willy or someone's bum . . ." He had to get away from it for a bit. "So I went off on my mountain bike. Actually, no . . . I went surfing for a couple of days."

Not long afterwards, this man asked to be transferred to another kind of police work. Both the researcher and I had a strong feeling that the research sessions played a part in allowing his defences against the disturbing and painful impact of this work to slowly break down. Perhaps he volunteered for the research because he sensed he needed a context to help him work this through. Whatever, the data from the sessions provide a rich picture of a worker poised on a kind of knife edge: on the one hand, almost always in touch with the emotional realities and forensic significance of what he is hearing—the denial, contradictions, deceit, self-deceit, the sudden effort to throw an interviewer off the scent—and, on the other, a man suffering from the damaging exposure to too much perversity and malevolence.

(4) The discovery of "complexity of particulars"

The closer we come to the raw emotional, relationship-based, turbulent, messy visceral data of practice, the more I think that the fact of the "complexity of particulars" forces itself on our attention. To really *understand* and capture in adequate concepts and formulations the character, meaning, and broader significance of the very specific people, families, organizational processes we are studying requires a terrific effort of emotional and methodological will-power. I have a special aversion to qualitative research in which lots of people are interviewed, and then the research is written up in loosely themed groupings of quotations from the research subjects. Any effort to interrogate the meaning of these utterances further is usually met with a defensive insistence that "What we have presented is what these people are telling us"—the unspoken part of the communication being, "So, bugger off with your clever interpretations, which are in fact your own oppressive distortions of these people's real experience which they have so generously shared."

Of course, there are very real and serious questions about how the research act can authentically capture the experience and meanings of the "other" without, as it were, engaging in an act of "othering". But I am clear that we desperately need our social work research to provide us with in-depth understanding of our complex psycho-social world. A key lesson from doing practice-near research is thus: *that each and every situation or context is unique and particular and must be understood—"apprehended"—in its own terms*. Its character or meaning cannot be "read off", or deduced, from some set of abstract principles.

I can now say a bit more about the bigger world view I suggest practice-near research partakes of: the dynamics shaping the everyday psycho-social world are *creative*, constantly combining elements of human capacities and functioning in original, new, unfamiliar ways to produce "complex particulars". Sometimes, this "creativity" is in the service of deadly and destructive ends—no two children are abused in exactly the same way. But, of course, this is not the end of the story—the strong family resemblances, or ingrained and repetitive patterns in human individual, group, organizational, or social life are not just the additive result of particulars that resemble one another being subsequently grouped by minds that recognize similarity. Patterns and resemblances must be the product of structuring, or patterning, or law-like principles at work somewhere. But these are what I think we have less idea about—though again it is possible to indicate where others have explored the territory (see chapter 14 for further exploration of this theme).

Anthony Giddens' theoretical work on how society is constituted and reproduces itself tried to create a space between sociological determinism and sociological individualism; neither absolute free "agency" of the social subject, nor total social structuring of the subject either. This resulted in his profound if clumsily named theory of "structuration" (Giddens, 1979, 1984). The critical realist post-Marxist philosophical tradition led by the work of Roy Bhaskar is another theoretical resource (Archer, Bhaskar, Collier, Lawson, & Norrie, 1998), articulating a kind of surface and depth model of social processes in which knowable social phenomena are produced by generative deep-structural principles.

Hearing the grass grow

> "If we had a keen vision and feeling of all ordinary human life, it would be like hearing the grass grow and the squirrel's heart beat and we should die of that roar which lies on the other side of silence."
>
> (George Eliot, *Middlemarch*, 1871)

The police constable presented earlier appeared to be gradually overcome by the roar that lies on the other side of silence. As for him, the dilemma of practice-near research reflects the predicament of social work in society—how much reality can we bear to know about? I suggested at the outset that a central social function of social work is both to disclose forms of suffering to society via engagement with them and, simultaneously, to protect society from too much painful awareness of the ugly facts that are constantly in our midst. I suppose someone might object that not all social work is as concerned with painful, ugly, perverse, toxic, intractable realities as I have painted it to be. This could be right, but my response would be that the easier bits of social work are perhaps not the ones that really need our urgent attention. If, as researchers, we do not have the courage to try to engage with the most unwelcome aspects of our professional task, then I think we are failing in our responsibilities to our practitioner colleagues. This reflects a more general conviction of mine that is no doubt recognizably psychoanalytic—that the power of the destructive and the negative is reduced or attenuated through fearless engagement with it and recognition of its nature; thereby we can be released into greater freedom, creativity, and even happiness. Often we cannot find the resources or courage to manage this, and so we tend to be condemned to repeat or hand on our miseries. Progress in human affairs may be slow but that does not mean it is not real, and that it does not need all our renewed efforts to sustain it. Good practice-near research is a contribution to this effort.

CHAPTER THIRTEEN

Front-line services, complexity, research, and policy

Introduction

There is a growing expectation in the public sector that the troubling and puzzling predicaments that present to policymakers, managers, and practitioners in mental health and social care should be understood through the application of knowledge derived from empirical research—on the model of the biomedical sciences—and that these predicaments should be responded to through interventions whose value and credibility has been assured through systematic evaluation. Commissioners of services rely increasingly on the evidence for the broad effectiveness, and cost-effectiveness, of psychotherapeutic interventions as treatments for specific problems (while trusting the pronouncements of the National Institute for Health and Care Excellence on the relative worth/significance of different forms of evidence).

Despite, or because of, this greater attention being paid to research findings as a source of clinical and policy decision making, there is

---

An earlier version of this chapter was published as A. Cooper & B. Wren, "Front-Line Services, Complexity, Research and Policy", *Psychoanalytic Psychotherapy, 26* (No. 3, 2012): 199–210.

still a concern that cutting-edge research of potential relevance to health and social care practitioners and the communities they serve takes too long to be "translated" into a usable form (e.g., Tansella & Thornicroft, 2009). To address this problem, innovative organizational structures known as Academic Health Sciences Centres (AHSCs) have been established across the UK. They are designed to enable the accelerated implementation of research findings in front-line settings, so that patient benefit- and health-improvements outcomes are delivered more rapidly.

It is argued that complexity in the relationships between research, clinical practice, and management is one key factor influencing this regrettable time-lag for research to move from bench to bedside. Hence, "complexity" is a central intellectual and operational variable to be tackled in pursuit of AHSCs' aims. To succeed, AHSCs must facilitate new kinds of relationships among these networks, guided by "implementation science" and cutting-edge policy analysis. Research on implementation means exploring any organizational and logistical difficulties in "applying experimental methods to service or policy change" (Craig et al., 2008), as well as identifying barriers to standardizing and delivering proven interventions and facilitating the creation of local strategies to overcome these barriers.

In this chapter we attempt a thoughtful response to these demands for the greater and more efficient application of research in our fields of mental health and social care. Coming from very different professional vantage points—systems thinking and critical psychology on the one hand, and psychoanalysis and social care on the other—we share a concern that a commitment to a biomechanical research programme will be of significant but limited value in our field. We are especially alarmed when mental ill health comes to be talked about as something located only "in" individuals, identified in terms of a specific aetiology, with treatment targeted at the individual impairment, and we question some of the assumptions of experimental research as the main research paradigm in mental health. We connect across different professional and disciplinary specialties to argue that the lived experience of front-line mental health work with adults and children is one of systemic complexity involving "index patients", family, kin, friendship and community networks, multi-professional and multi-agency involvement, and quite often the legal system. We fear that the AHSC model will under-represent these crucial sites of "complexity" in the overall research picture if a more deterministic model of causality is espoused.

The task of developing a better understanding of the difficulties of clients in mental health and social care and offering them more effective services will not be tackled simply by more formidable research–practitioner–community partnerships, unless there is a sophisticated grasp of how the target difficulties in mental health emerge and evolve across time and context.

Complexity: a simple example

Here is a simple example of "complexity" in the area of mental health: a woman with a diagnosis of bipolar disorder finds a partner with a diagnosis of schizophrenia. When they are both "well", things go pretty well for them, and better than before. When one of them is less well, it also destabilizes the other, who in turn further destabilizes the first. Neither of them has much capacity to "contain" the disturbance of the other. In addition the woman has her 12-year-old son staying with her at weekends, and their relationship can at times be confrontational; arguments seem to be worse when mother's partner is present. The nature of this "system" is both psychodynamic and, well, systemic. Moreover, the adults live within separate health and social care delivery systems, and their key workers don't always see eye to eye. One is more psychoanalytic in her thinking, and the other more cognitive-behavioural. Sometimes they proffer advice or set up interventions that are in some tension with one another. Statutory review processes are slightly different and run to different time scales in the two areas.

Embracing complexity, not controlling it

Few would seriously suggest that this plausible (fictional) situation has no bearing on the mental health "outcomes" of each person. Equally, the relationship between the two patients and the child neither fully explains their "poor mental health" nor holds out the hope of a "cure" for either or both of them. It is just one "reality factor" in their total mental health picture. The anxious rational policymaker might decide on a new system of cross-agency protocols to address the system tensions in cases such as these. It might do some good, but it would also be a further systemic intervention in an already complex picture, so it will contribute its own new feedback effects and probably generate new unintended consequences. Interventions implemented in complex systems are likely to have diverse, far-reaching, and non-linear effects.

Meanwhile, the anxious traditional researcher might design a randomized controlled trial (RCT) to test for the best intervention for a bipolar sufferer. Acknowledging that being in relationship with someone who has a major mental health diagnosis complicates the causal picture with respect to the independent variable—the treatment—she might be wise to exclude people with social relationships with other mental health sufferers.

In trying to predict the outcome of a particular therapeutic intervention, it is impossible for the researcher to measure all the variables believed to be actual or possible influences on the problem; furthermore, there are "chance" factors at work about which little or nothing may be known. If what we want from research is generalizable knowledge, then we cannot elucidate all the factors whose occurrence, or failure to occur, might actually contribute to a particular outcome with respect to one sufferer. Complex chains of events in their particularity cannot be subsumed under generalizable laws (Lieberson, 1997). Furthermore, pathways in such complex systems are often non-linear; the causal factors affecting a set of circumstances may be interactive and not just additive. So the best we can do is conceptualize the likely outcomes in broad probabilistic terms, providing a very limited idea about what will be the mental health trajectory of any one patient and what approach is likely to be helpful.

Indeed, in mental health and social care practice, many of our key research and clinical questions require the unravelling of complex probabilistically linked chains of events, rather than simply searching for the cause or causes of some phenomenon of interest, or the outcome of an intervention. Recent published work on child protection and complexity invokes notions of "indicative" predictability (Stevens & Cox, 2008) rather than absolute predictability, and *The Munro Review of Child Protection* (2011a) is notable as the first major British policy document to embrace systemic complexity as a central theoretical principle shaping a specific domain of policy analysis.

The traditional researcher might do research that does tell us *something* useful about cases like the one described, but a great deal less than we want to know (or could know) about the lived realities of our patients, and how best to help them—at either a clinical or a policy level. Well, you may think, "Better to know something useful that has been properly researched" than to be left with just "complexity", fumbling along with our accumulated practice wisdom, clinical experience, and faulty professional judgement. But is this the only alternative? Can complexity be researched?

Can research and policymaking, rather than attempting to eliminate or reduce complexity, embrace it and work with it as a necessary feature of social and personal reality? How we answer depends on what we mean by "complexity" and how it differs from "unnecessarily complicated". Modern theoretical perspectives on complexity in all realms of life and the sciences argue that complexity is an inherent feature of how our worlds are constituted.

A philosophical note: what does "complexity" mean?

Complexity means more than just "complicated" or "comprising many variables", and more than "too involved and unpredictable to understand and research". It has important implications for the kinds of research we consider relevant to influencing people's lives, and it entails a shift in our generally accepted ideas of how causes and effects are related. In turn, this has implications for appropriate models of research and for the science → research → policy → treatment → service design chain.

Complexity assumes that the causal factors affecting a set of circumstances may be interactive and not just additive. While additive relationships can be decomposed so that the causal powers of parts can be separately examined and researched, interactive relationships generate new, "emergent" properties in systems or states of affairs that are not reducible to the component elements, although they are dependent upon them. Emergent properties of systems are often not fully or even partly predictable. The same set of basic elements may generate quite different emergent properties as a result of tiny fluctuations in one or more elements. In non-linear systems, small differences in initial conditions can produce very different outcomes; this is called "sensitive dependence on initial conditions".

The nature of the "laws" governing the production and development of complex systems is thus different from the standard conception of "scientific law", which assumes law to be exceptionless and universal. It is now widely accepted in the philosophy of science (although not by scientists wedded to traditional methodologies) that the objects of study of very few domains of scientific investigation conform to the "standard model" of scientific law—or, at least, that science deploying the standard model will only "capture" a partial picture of both the nature of the object and its principles of development. The picture it does capture is not completely wrong, just selective and limited (Mitchell, 2009).

Many, and possibly all, of the "domains of investigation" of science are not governed by universal or timeless laws, but are the result of accidents of historical development with laws to match. This may even be true of the laws of the physical universe we inhabit—the physical laws we know may be just one set among many that are logically possible, but not "actualized". This is almost certainly true of the "laws" of chemistry, and even more so of biological laws. At each level, the nature of the universe we do inhabit constrains but does not determine the domain of laws at the next level. Thus, the laws of chemistry cannot contradict the laws of physics, but they are not determined by them. Our chemical universe could have been different.

Chemistry, biology, genetics, brain development are all separate domains of complexity. We accept that they are implicated in human development and thus in the production of "mental health" and mental "ill health". Psychology and social relationships are also domains of complexity and can also be seen as more or less governed by their own variety of "laws" or "law-like" principles. The further we move from physics in the direction of human psychological, social, political and economic development, and behaviour, the less "stable", permanent, exceptionless is the nature of the system of "laws" governing the domain of inquiry, and the more does "predictability" of the conventional kind recede. This does not mean that chaos or complete randomness is the result. But the nature of the more or less stable "patterning" or "lawfulness" of these complex systems does become harder to ascertain and describe with confidence.

Another complexity factor is that meanings and relationships are part of the picture too. Are they aspects of a total "causal" picture? Or are they something quite different—a separate order of existence? Philosophers have worried about this since the dawn of time. We take the view that they are both. Meanings (symbolic systems, constructs, theories, frames of reference, stories, narratives, and so forth) are real, different from billiard balls, but perfectly capable of interacting (causally) with billiard balls. After all, a billiard ball is only a billiard ball rather than a spherical lump of coloured matter because someone invented the game of billiards—which was an act of imagination. Matter would probably never have assumed billiard-ball form in the history of the universe had this act of imagination not occurred.

And finally (for the purposes of this chapter), an additional level of complexity is the fact of the interaction among these various levels or domains of complexity in the generation of something as familiar to us as "a depressive episode" or "a risk of breakdown" or "a risk of child maltreatment".

Mental health work and complexity

The fact of mental health being a site for the operation of complex, multi-level, feedback-laden processes poses a number of overlapping issues for debate by those who design research in mental health and those who have authority for policy decisions. Understanding our field as complex involves a rejection of the idea of mental ill health as something located only "in" individuals. A prevailing, if not universal, model of mental well-being and illness is that these are significantly generated ("caused") by relationships at many levels, with developmental processes (individual, family, professional, community, political) as a key dimension. The recipient of a mental health service may ostensibly be the individual, but the individual is understood to belong in a complex nexus of relationships (sibling–sibling, husband–wife, pupil–teacher). And, of course, families, schools and communities are emergent and historically contextualized systems, composed of more than the sum of their individual parts. Yet in contemporary mental health research, there is a constant expansion of linear-science-based understandings of individual pathologies, and it is important for health policy and service development to recognize that clinical procedures founded in such understandings will be limited in their effectiveness.

In context-rich causal scenarios, two kinds of factors typically come together to produce outcomes of real interest: (1) factors that have traditionally been allocated the role of cause (like genes or faulty cognitions) and (2) factors that traditionally have not been a focus for research but, rather, relegated to the general amorphous context or background "noise" (such as the social environment). Most psychological problems share this multi-level, multi-component profile. The challenge for policymakers is to find how many small explanations fit together.

Furthermore, even when these layers of relationship are taken into account and included in the "complexity diagram", there are further issues to consider. Relationships are organized by "meanings"—unconscious, co-constructed, systemic—and so a new language enters the picture that is harder to capture within a "hard systems" paradigm, even if these same systems are posited as complex and adaptive. A focus on meaning implies a concern with people's representations of reality, their understanding of their lives, their past, and their relationships. It also implies an acknowledgment that people are active in trying to make sense of their experience and the behaviour of themselves and others. This reflexive aspect of human thinking creates further uncertainties for those trying to understand processes in mental health research and treatment.[1]

A sophisticated psycho-social approach to mental health is founded on the idea of complex feedback-laden causes. It is helpful to consider the analogy of different understandings of the aetiology of tuberculosis (see Byrne, 1998). A reductionist account describes the exposure of a susceptible individual to infection and the consequent development of the clinical disease in that individual. A *social* account in epidemiology may involve a description of the result of the aggregate of individual cases. Or we can go beyond this to a complex account of the genesis of individual cases in terms of diet, housing conditions, and ethnicity. For a truly "complex" model, however, we have to think of the *interaction* of the system levels. TB is a disease of societies that are highly unequal. The re-emergence of TB in New York in the 1990s, for example, was not just a consequence of AIDS, as a contingent factor. AIDS itself is a complex social product (given that shared needle use is one of its causes—a consequence of social alienation among the young). Add in the interactive effects of home overcrowding (due to increases in housing costs) and the relative collapse of free public health and hospital care, and you have a multi-system, multi-level interactive account of complex causality.

The experimental paradigm in mental health research

While we acknowledge that some aspects of classical empirical science offer power and rigour to researchers, we question whether the traditional hypothesis-testing experimental paradigm is well-suited to analysing causal complexity. As Mitchell (2009) argues, in the fields of psychiatry and psychology we are aware of a "deep" uncertainty that is not adequately researched by methods better suited to more certain, predictable, and static parts of nature.

Indeed, it is striking that the RCT, with its clear methodological and statistical procedures for ensuring rigour, has been granted a foremost role in the search for knowledge about causal processes and structures in our field, given widespread concerns that the findings from RCT's may offer neither clinical generalizability nor genuine scientific advance. This is partly because experimental research in psychology seems to have settled into a rigid set of practices, rituals, and unexamined assumptions (e.g., Costall, 2010).[2] Controlled experimental research assumes that causes are simple, and that everything except the supposed cause, and the effect of that cause, can be held constant—even though in research on complex phenomena, the "independent variables" are neither strictly distinct nor uncontaminated. Additionally, such research makes every attempt to neutralize the effects of human volition, even though the "interventions" being evaluated (e.g., forms of psychotherapy) may be active, not passive. The statistical methods (like regression analysis), which aim to account for the action of several possible causes, assume additivity and linearity, rather than interaction and complexity.

Ultimately, the work required to detect the lawful relations in nonlinear systems is well beyond what can be accessed by hypothesis-testing experimental research. The quantitative methods able to map likely future pathways and trajectories in complex systems are still in their infancy. There are techniques like "fuzzy-set analysis" (e.g., Ragin, 2008) that pay close attention to cases as configurations, and to the different combinations of causally relevant conditions linked to an outcome. Furthermore, we consider that it is still respectable to build general knowledge from case-oriented research, from understandings of specific cases in specific contexts, and from studying cases holistically in projects that require a close, detailed reading of rich and extensive data—for example, from transcripts of clinical work, disciplined observation, focus groups, and interviews.

One of the problems with controlled experimental research is that it assumes a characteristic and very particular kind of perspective-free *objectivity* that aims to minimize all the subjectivity of the researcher. This is objectivity that aspires to "knowledge that bears no trace of the knower—knowledge unmarked by prejudice or skill, fantasy or judgment, wishing or striving" (Daston & Galison, 2007, p. 17). In clinical trials, such objectivity is supposedly ensured, and researcher subjectivity kept at bay, by procedures like the manualization of interventions and the "blinding" of researcher who rates participants at different stages of treatment. Daston and Galison (2007) speak of the distinct qualities associated with objectivity—certainty, truth, precision, replicability, suppression of the scientist's will—and note that these are more than just competences. They can be thought of as "epistemic virtues" that must be preached and practised in order for the scientist to know the world. Allegiance to these values and their associated practices constitutes a way of scientific life. In the complex world of psychotherapy where the knowing self is a precondition of knowledge, not an obstacle to it, these are questionable assumptions indeed.

Science, non-science, and professional judgement

Increasingly in public health, researchers are widely presented as the new aristocracy. The idea of research as the chief, unproblematic source of knowledge for clinical policy decisions assumes a pragmatic, non-ideological, approach to public policy, surely at odds with other indicators that vested interests often dominate the field of policy. This apparent veneration of research evidence is often coupled with a suspicion of professional practice and power, and the undermining of the value of professional judgement, which is increasingly seen as highly partial, anecdotal, and arbitrary. It is difficult in the current climate to take a position of challenging the primacy of science over other forms of knowing. Yet investigations into the history of scientific endeavour show it to be a history of success and failure, of politics and ideology. Science is enormously enriched by *un*scientific methods and *un*scientific results, while procedures and results that have often been regarded as essential parts of the scientific endeavour are quietly set aside or circumvented (Feyerabend, 1975).

Over the last fifty years in the natural and human sciences (including psychology, economics, and political theory), there has been a noticeable move away from the self-critical exercise of judgement in favour of algorithmic rules of rationality. Such suspicion of trained judgement in fact misconstrues the scientific method and caricatures the nature of informed decision making. Expert decision making is a rapid, intuitive, and seemingly idiosyncratic process that incorporates and makes sense of multiple and complex data elements, including subtle contextual evidence. This is in contrast to novice decision making which tends to be formulaic, rigid, and rule-bound. We would wish to resist the eclipse of the kind of tacit knowledge which is demonstrated in the exercise of active, well-honed, clinical judgement by experienced and competent clinicians, drawing on great familiarity with the material as well as on other forms of relevant knowledge.

An outline model for complexity research

Returning to our brief case example, how might we develop a research study that embraces complexity but also advances our understanding of practice efficacy in a systematic manner? What principles would inform our design?

Practitioner research using small cohorts or even single cases typically generates its research questions from "clinical hunches"—experientially derived intuitions about "what worked" (or didn't) in the course of an intervention; what change processes occurred across time in relation to the intervention; what factors in a complex picture may have promoted or prevented change, destabilization, impasse, deterioration; and so on. Such hunches can inform either retrospective or prospective designs and be oriented either to the investigation of specific "causal" dimensions of complex clinical processes or to the descriptive elucidation of the interaction of multiple factors in producing outcomes and typical patterns of system behaviour. Several methodological principles are at work in even this rather simple characterization.

First, the point of departure is naturalistic. Because ordinary psycho-social phenomena are generated through complexity dynamics, no two sets of circumstances will be identical. However, strong "family resemblances" among phenomena, or selected dimensions of phenomena (such as case networks involving intimate relationships between people with major mental illnesses), will be a valid and important object of research. This idea is similar to that of "demi-regs" (relatively stable, recurring, but not universal regularities in the patterns of social life). The research "problem" makes itself known through practice experience, and the context of "discovery" is set by such experience. One does not attempt to control out "extraneous" variables; rather, they must be explicitly factored in because it is the interaction between the "variable" of special interest and the total context that *is* the research focus. The study takes a group of "real" phenomena, encountered naturalistically, as its object. The best approximation to research design of the kind we advocate is in Pawson and Tilley's (1997) *Realistic Evaluation*; these authors advocate for "applied research with its ensuing and decidedly concrete task of discovering what works for whom in a set of *given* circumstances" (p. 86).

Second, the study will take place across time—not because we are especially interested in "outcomes", but because complex systems evolve, and they fluctuate, in how near or far they are from "equilibrium"; understanding the dynamics of these is the route to "knowing" the nature of the system, including what interventions, gestures, or contextual adjustments might improve the quality of life of key system members. Charting system change and stability through time potentially reveals the underlying or deep patterning at work which explains "stability", as well as dynamics associated with disequilibrium, phase transitions, and other relatively enduring changes of system state.

Third, the study will probably best deploy a cross-case comparative methodology because we are interested to understand both the particularity or unique character of each system and the "pattern that connects" different but similar system instances into a "family", always remembering that such networks of similarity will have fuzzy rather than rigid boundaries.

So, a hypothetical nine-month-long study of six case networks involving partnered subjects, with both partners having a diagnosis of major mental illness, might yield findings such as:

» Permanent or temporary separations between two such people sometimes improves the overall mental health of one or both, and sometimes not.

» The reciprocally interacting fluctuations of state characteristic of an "unstable" couple are, in some cases, less damaging to their overall functioning than permanent separations, and sometimes not.

» "Couple-focused" casework in such cases appears to work much better when the caseworkers are professionally compatible.

» A range of occurrences identified in the course of the study—adverse life events affecting the individual service-users, interruptions to the stability of services provided, changes in benefit status and so on—were a significant trigger for relationship instability.

These findings are characteristic for *an open complex human system*. The "variable" of supposed primary interest—partnerships between two adults with major mental health problems—emerges as *one factor of significance* that does confer upon the total system of which they are a part a set of distinctive qualities, setting such systems apart, but only a little, from comparable systems without this feature. The couple relationship is not a closed system, and isolating it for "controlled study" is, in fact, a waste of time—and of public money. But much of practical and ethical value can be learned and applied from a study of the kind imagined here, assuming that those learning from it are receptive to thinking about their work in terms of complex systems rather than additive, mechanical ones.

Thus, the "theoretically driven" nature of the practice → research → interventions → policy → service development project comes full circle, though modified to reflect the discussion here.

Concluding remarks

To make reasonable policy decisions in the fields of mental health and social care, we need to debate very seriously the way evidence accumulates and is pieced together. Policy decisions are not derived in any straightforward way from research or from rule-governed meta-analyses of research. Policy is "theory incarnate" (Pawson, 2006). Interventions are theories too—theories about how to change thinking and behaviour. There is much work to be done in working out how we best "juxtapose, adjudicate, reconcile, consolidate and situate evidence" (Pawson, 2006) within and between theoretical models—whether "systemic", psychodynamic, or more broadly "psycho-social"—drawing on findings from neuroscience, developmental psychology, genetics, evolutionary theory, social science, philosophy, and ethics. But policy that is governed by a view of how psychological and social reality works based on "standard" assumptions about causes and effects and predictability will be severely restricted in its impact. It may even generate more confusion than it clears up—what are sometimes referred to as "unintended consequences"—because it will be an intervention in a set of systems that are much more sophisticated in their nature than are the models of reality driving the research and the interventions that come along to try to "improve things".

Because these "mistaken" models and practices are not *wholly* mistaken, there will probably be some beneficial impact. The partial success of evidence-based interventions leads researchers and policymakers to redouble their efforts at improving the success rate, but deploying the same paradigms of investigation.[3] Research implementation requires a more powerful understanding of causality.

In doing psychotherapy responsibly, we draw on a whole range of resources—personal resonances, theoretical concepts and research-based knowledge, ethical awareness, and political sensibility. Policymakers need to recognize that the way this extraordinarily complex interweaving of sources of knowledge and understanding is done involves a particular awareness of the relationship between particulars and universals, developing a repertoire of understanding with which to help make sense of the "complex particulars" we work with. Clinicians rely on both "generalized knowledge"—to provide a framework for observing our clients, feeling and interacting with them and making sense of their stories—and a sense of how each family, individual, network, and so on is unique in its own way and has to be understood and "known" for itself because it is a creative outcome of "complexity". This relationship is different from that between a sample and an individual, which assumes that if we had a complete "sample" we would have absolute knowledge; we would not, because the relationships are not additive/linear.

The human world and our knowledge of it are highly dynamic, and we need conceptual frameworks to accommodate contingency, dynamic robustness, and "deep" uncertainty. Complexity science recognizes that in the human sciences there are no inevitable outcomes, no linear laws, no single answers. It is non-reductionist and rejects the theory of levels (the proposition that the simpler can explain the more complex). Complexity can guide us towards purposeful action—but we have to know a lot and be able to manage what we know in new ways. Yet we do believe we can carry out, and draw on, research to try to understand what a possible set of outcomes might be and—in sites of robust complexity—intervene in order to achieve what we want to see happen, even in the knowledge that many further explanatory possibilities remain untapped.

Notes

1. As Byrne (1998) notes, the administration of placebos in clinical trials of drugs is the tribute reductionist, simple linear science pays to the reflexive capacities of human beings.

2. These include the use of large numbers of "subjects", the use of standardized measures, the disregard of other aspects of the data that might be of interest, the almost exclusive focus on averages, and the reverence for the 0.05 *p*-value cut-off.

3. The situation is analogous to that described by Kuhn in *The Structure of Scientific Revolutions* (1975). There was an astronomical observation called "the anomalous perihelion of Mercury" that simply did not fit with the rest of the theory that (satisfactorily) explained the functioning of the solar system. Scientists postulated many varieties of as-yet-undiscovered cause that, had one of them been true, would have assimilated this anomaly into the existing theory. But when Einstein came along with his new theory of space–time–matter, the perihelion of Mercury was no longer "anomalous": it was predicted by the theory. The new theory was more inclusive, and subsumed the old one as adequate to account for particular cases or degrees of sensitivity of observation. So it had been partly right, not wholly wrong.

CHAPTER FOURTEEN

Entering the underworld: unconscious life and the research process

Introduction

Psycho-social and psychoanalytic research is interested in "researching beneath the surface" of individual experience and social relationships in the context of professional social work, social care practice, and clinical and therapeutic work of all kinds (Clarke & Hoggett, 2009). But what exactly does this mean? And how do you set about doing it? What faculties and skills are involved? How can we be sure of our methodological ground in this endeavour? What are some of the things we have discovered through this endeavour? These are some of the questions I engage with in this chapter. Most of the live research material in this chapter is drawn from work with, or the work of, doctoral students on the Professional Doctorates in Social Work and Social Care at the Tavistock. The process of generating a distinctive psychoanalytic method of research owes as much if not more to them, and their deep engagement with the research process, than it does to me.

The notion of "entering the underworld" is double-edged. Many of the projects undertaken by social work and social care doctoral researchers at the Tavistock give some voice and recognition both to populations of vulnerable, marginalized, disempowered people and, similarly, to dimensions of professional experience that lie outside the reach of our familiar theoretical and practice discourses. The research methods we use to access and articulate these experiences involve an engagement with both the social and individual unconscious lives of these populations, ourselves as professionals, and the social field occupied by social work itself. How we try to do this is one main themes of this chapter. But qualitative data analysis must proceed in some "orderly" and systematic way, and it cannot just be an exercise in free association to the material. So, many researchers opt for some form of inductive data-analytic strategy, alongside the psychoanalytic engagement, when tackling the mass of material their projects generate. The principles of Grounded Theory, Thematic Analysis, and Interpretive Phenomenological Analysis are all varieties of essentially inductive approaches that reduce the data to small manageable components and then proceed to link them together and build a broader conceptual picture using various methods of coding. A psychoanalytic approach to the data is neither primarily inductive nor deductive in my view, but interpretive. How such "interpretation" can work is the main theme of this chapter. The more technical question of how to link interpretations of the data to a systematic analysis of texts is a topic for another book.

To enable the reader to begin to share something of the experiences I want to describe and explore, I start with a joke:

> "Why do you bury a social worker at 600 feet?
> Because, deep down they're really good people."

This joke is one among many gathered by a doctoral student as part of his research into social work and humour (Jordan, 2015). It serves well, for a number of reasons, as a starting point for this chapter's exploration although, in order to say why, I need to deconstruct its humorous impact and reveal some of its more morbid components. I hope an appreciation of these can yield up both a metaphor that helps articulate the distinctive nature of the research programme that has emerged at the Tavistock over the last ten years, a deepening of the meaning of "surface and depth" in research processes, and also signal something about the ideological tendencies of this work and its contribution to helping us think about the place of social work in our society.

How deep?

So, why *do* you bury a social worker at 600 feet? Not six feet you notice, but six hundred—six feet under being far too close, too near the surface for comfort or safety, presumably. Down a mine shaft, that's how deep they need to go. Of course, the punchline discloses in disguised form the reason why: dead and buried they're safely reunited with their deeply buried compassionate natures; alive and kicking they're something else—dangerous, bad, despite themselves it seems. "The only really good social worker is a dead social worker" appears to be *the* message. Or one message, because, like most sophisticated humour, the joke captures and condenses a set of contradictory currents of thought and feeling and plays them one against another.

The punchline speaks to an anxiety about the dangerousness or perhaps the deadliness of the living social worker, but simultaneously it rescues us from a corresponding anxiety about our murderous hostility to this figure by evoking an affirming cliché—"deep down, they're really ok". The social worker is thus concurrently condemned and then redeemed. The cliché works on us in another register. I think, evoking an equally clichéd image of a soft, woolly liberal mindset often attributed to social workers, always prepared to excuse, redeem, forgive, explain away, understand the worst aspects of people's behaviour towards others; a mindset often invoked to account for social workers' alleged propensity for indecision, inaction, failure to look harsh realities in the face. In turn, this stereotype is playing against its antithesis, the image of the powerful, destructive, intrusive wrecker of lives and relationships, a source of such anxiety that even death and an ordinary decent burial are insufficient to alleviate our fears.

On this reading, the joke brings to the surface, in an acceptable and highly condensed form, a complex network of ambivalent currents of feeling about social workers, and about social work—and then, I would suggest, buries them again. The relief we gain from engaging with the joke is real, but transitory, fleeting. A joke like this *can* be a point of departure for real thinking, and it certainly embodies the complexity of real and serious thought, but you have to work hard to locate what this consists of.

Social work (as we are all too aware) is a profoundly ambivalently positioned and valued activity socially. Why? Well surely because we constantly threaten to "bring to the surface"—bring to mind—news of deeply disturbing and painful truths and realities about the lives and predicaments of people in our social midst who are suffering, dying needlessly, traumatized, traumatizing, displaced, abused, abusing, neglected, neglectful. And what of the social workers themselves? We too cannot be immune from ambivalence about the painfulness and disturbance bound up in the daily task. In Stephen Jordan's research, jokes and humour are research data, the basis of a serious investigation, but you cannot, unfortunately, write a doctorate just by compiling a list of jokes. Interrogating, analysing, mining data for its unconscious contents is really hard work, a process that usually involves engaging with discomforting feelings and thoughts if it is to be really productive.

In at the deep end

How does this work in practice? I shall describe a process that unfolded in the course of a two-hour research seminar with three doctoral students at varying stages of their respective projects. The seminar begins with Kathleen discussing her analysis of one lengthy narrative interview with a man who has had testicular cancer. Her project aims to understand and conceptualize the "psycho-social anxieties" of fathers who have had this illness and, in particular, to look at their relationships with their sons (Russell, 2015). There seems to be a well-established increased risk factor for the sons of fathers who have this diagnosis.

Kathleen is interested in tracing what kinds of anxieties the illness mobilized in these men, how they experienced and managed their anxieties for themselves and in relation to others including medical staff, as well as how the medical environment seems to have responded in turn. She is deploying Hollway and Jefferson's (2012) notion of "defended subjects" in her approach to her data, but also using the principles of Interpretative Phenomenological Analysis (IPA) to assist her in systematically trawling the transcripts.

On this day, as she talks about the process, she refers two or three times, rapidly and in passing, to the fact that of the ten men she interviewed, this was the one "she really did not like" for some reason. She refers to how, in his interview, he seemed very critical of doctors, and especially women doctors; how he had seemed disparaging of his own wife; how she had travelled to his home to conduct the interview on an afternoon when heavy snow started. She had expected the interview to last about two hours, but it had taken three and a half. The subject had shown no awareness of her possible situation, and she had come to feel uncomfortably trapped. There are many powerful vignettes in the subject's long interview. One involved his angry recollection of having his genitalia examined by a female doctor who had not used the latex gloves medical staff usually put on when conducting physical examinations. Finally Kathleen says, "But I think I need to put aside that feeling of dislike, that's something about me, it belongs in therapy or somewhere . . . I think I need to try to concentrate on analysing the transcript."

I have the advantage in this seminar of knowing this data a bit better than any of the other participants (apart from Kathleen!), and I decide to punctuate the discussion at this point. I wasn't so sure about this distinction Kathleen has just constructed, and I suggest that maybe we can't be so sure that excluding Kathleen's feeling of dislike for her research subject from the field of analysis is helpful. Maybe, in fact, it can tells us something, deepen our understanding of the material?

Using a simple technique familiar to us from many varieties of training, I suggest that Kathleen is quiet for a while and lets the rest of the group free-associate to, and think about, what they have heard so far. The themes or hypotheses that emerge in discussion are as follows:

- The man appears to be afflicted by deep anxieties about injury/ damage to his masculinity' or "manhood".
- Some of his material evoked images of a tiny dependent baby, at the mercy of a carer/mother who must tend, clean, care for his genitals.
- His hostility to doctors and carers seems to be linked to a strong sense of not being in control. They, not he, are in control and they are "getting it wrong".
- His complaint about the woman doctor who did not wear protective gloves can be read as a metaphor for his own fears about intimate exposure to the powerful woman/carer. He wanted a barrier or defence against her in place.
- In turn, this might alert us to his conflicted feelings about the interview itself. He is voluntarily "exposing" his anxieties and fears to Kathleen, but also feels very anxious about doing so. Kathleen picks up his hostility to "women" but perhaps also more directly to herself? He subtly controls her and makes her feel trapped.
- Might we be thinking here about a *particular* constellation of anxieties, present in some men, in which their genitals are both a site of anxiety but also of gendered/ sexualized control?

Thought about in this way, a focus on Kathleen's own subjective experience of the interview potentially deepens and confirms the validity of formulations or hypotheses derived more straightforwardly from the interview text itself. Her "dislike" of the subject may not be just "her stuff", but a countertransference experience, related to his very conflicted, ambivalent relationship to her. As such we do not judge it—after all, this is merely one familiar form that defences against anxiety can take.

Our project is less ambitious: to try to *describe,* in as much psychological and social depth as we can, a particular subject's emotionally complex response to an intensely anxiety-provoking (though normally not in fact life-threatening) illness, *as it emerges in the live material of the research interview.* The key transference and countertransference elements of the interview are located not "in the material" but in the relationship between researcher and interviewee, including the way the researcher's own defences are mobilized. To decode these processes requires other psychoanalytically attuned research minds. This idea is presented in a more abstract form in Chapter 15.

The coffee break

After this discussion, we break for coffee. Two students including Kathleen leave the room, leaving me, my co-tutor, and one student, Nancy. I ask Nancy how she is, and she replies that she is fine, but very bound up with the birth of her first grandchild just a couple of weeks ago. She shows us photos of him, and we exchange stories and reminiscences of our memories of our children's early infancy. I become momentarily weepy, recalling the first photograph I saw of my adopted son when he was 3 days old, and how his eyes seemed to look straight into the camera—at me. My co-tutor then leaves the room. Nancy now tells me about something different—the intense pain and conflict she has experienced in relation to her grandson being circumcised a week ago. She describes how, with her own sons, she could not "look" but, as a grandmother, had decided she should look and bear witness. She says, "It felt like a terrible act of mutilation", and she continues by telling of the care and attention the tiny baby's genitals have needed over the last week. I comment briefly on how close all this is to what we've just been discussing.

The rest of the seminar group returns. I think to myself, "There's something going on here", and I ask Nancy whether it's ok to replay some of the conversation we've just had. She says it's fine. After the others have heard, one member of the group ponders on whether the experience of circumcision is "remembered", carried within adult circumcised men as some kind of embodied trauma. Suddenly Kathleen sits up and says, "My God, I've just remembered that this man we were discussing is Jewish."

Where are we now? What have we learned or discovered? It's hard to know exactly, but I think we all felt and believed that somehow as a group we had achieved a much deeper, more immediate and "alive" emotional contact with the research material in question. At the time, the seminar process did not feel to me dangerous, or risky—I think we are all pretty accustomed to the surprises, shocks, sudden connections that occur when we allow "free association" to take its course in working on research material in this way. But as I wrote this up, it did begin to feel risky, in the sense that I felt we had entered "taboo territory" and that the material I am narrating is probably evoking strong emotional responses in readers. There are certainly no definitive, concrete "findings" to be distilled from this process, but entering this kind of conflicted, intimate, emotional, and cultural territory can mobilize anxiety about (among others) the sort of "wild" inferences that could (in the wrong hands) be made.

So what is the nature of this territory? A short account of the rest of this seminar offers one kind of answer.

In the dream space?

Another student, Katharine, now picks up the running with an account of her recent preparations towards writing her registration document. She intends to research the lived experience of ordinary front-line social care worker staff who work with dying people and to relate this to the current "End of Life Care Strategy" policy. She has been observing training sessions for care staff arising from local implementation of this new policy. She describes becoming aware of a whole range of professional systems for dealing with death, and how these often seem to impede one another—GPs who seem to delay signing death certificates for inexplicable reasons, ambulance services that only respond under prescribed circumstances to the need to remove corpses, and very difficult medical conditions encountered in ordinary care settings that make "managing dying with dignity" a near-impossible task.

Katharine describes moving between this observational work, her day job and her private life and comments that she sometimes feels as though she is in contact with a kind of "underworld". We clarify that for her this "underworld" means the world of death and its management.

But perhaps the whole seminar has entered a kind of underworld—of emotionally intense experiences and relationships and processes that are not commonly, or easily, spoken about? I say to the seminar that perhaps it is a kind of "dream space"—a realm of social existence that is active all the time but is just beneath conscious or surface social awareness and even discourse. Our awareness or knowledge of death is "half knowledge": death is something we know "about" but usually don't think about in an emotionally engaged way.

Another member of the course group described shortly after these events how she had been speaking the previous day with a young person who is looked after. He had been talking about child abuse and said, "It's not hidden, it's there to be seen if only people will look." This pretty much describes the way I think about the nature of unconscious processes in individuals, in groups, in institutions, and in society. Clinically, it is a view best described and elaborated by the American psychoanalyst Thomas Ogden:

> The unconscious is not "subconscious"; it is an aspect of the indivisible totality of consciousness. Similarly meaning (including unconscious meaning) is *in* the language being used, not under or behind it. Freud [1915e] believed the term "subconscious" to be "incorrect and misleading" since the Unconscious does not lie "under" consciousness. [Ogden, 1999, p. 215]

For Ogden and the clinical theorists on whom he draws, psychoanalytic work is conducted in a "field", created by the meeting of two or more people who bring into their relationship their unconscious life. The interplay of unconscious processes between them creates a new phenomenon—he calls it the analytic "third", which is dependent on these two contributors but is itself not entirely reducible to its two component parts. It has its own creativity and generativity. Organizational consultants and theorists in the Tavistock tradition, such as David Armstrong, essentially think of institutions in much the same way. For myself, I believe that societies and social relationships are also inherently constituted in and through their unconscious dimension, although they cannot be simply reduced to this. A social "field" is also a field of unconscious relationships and processes.

And so, if we broadly accept Freud's ideas about jokes and humour as communications that are structured according to the same principles as dreams, the joke about social workers represents a communication both about how social work is positioned in this field, at the same time as it emanates from the dynamic workings of this field. It is a momentary point of entry into this social "underworld" where social workers are (in phantasy) killed and buried as deep down as they can be. But as we know, during periods of social crisis surrounding the kinds of work we do—usually but not always triggered by the death of a child—these phantasies can assume all too "real" a manifestation.

Mental pain and research data: a narrative interview

Many of the projects informing this chapter deployed free-narrative interviewing methods (Hollway & Jefferson, 2012), which were then analysed using a blend of thematic analysis and psychoanalytically informed attention to the emotional dynamics of the researcher–participant encounter, as well as the textual evidence for unconscious process. This section of the chapter illustrates some of the qualities of emotional immediacy and pain that the interview method can elicit, and it then moves to consider a higher order research methodological problem: how to find the cross-cutting meaning or sense embedded in a cluster of qualitative interviews which might yield up a more general hypothesis or concept that unifies the data field.

The researcher, Dr Raelton Gibbs, is also a Major in the Salvation Army, and his project centred around five lengthy biographical narrative interviews with residents of Salvation Army hostels for homeless people (Gibbs, 2013). His project transpired to be quite simple in one sense: an effort to really listen to the biographical and emotional histories that a few typical residents of these hostels narrated when given the opportunity. Not particularly ambitious, one might think—but I wonder how many among us have ever really given serious thought to what the life stories of long-term homeless people are about? As it turns out, few people anywhere have given this serious documented attention. Raelton did generate more complex conceptual findings from his study, and I shall come to these a little later. But to get us started, here is a short extract from the beginning of one of his narrative interviews:

(RG) Ok so er if I can ask you please tell me your life story and all the events.

(A) Life story, including back home?

(RG) And personally up till now, and start where ever you like and take as much time as you want.

(A) I am originally an ethnic from Somalia, and and we were about, I mean brothers my eldest brother Adam is dead already they shot him in front of me and er my second sister Sophia she used to be as a manager at our restaurant eh in Mogadishu I am the third and my brother is Rod his name is my youngest brother and my dad and my mum that means we were 6 all of us.

And er we had a minibus the one who used to work for the public service in Mogadishu and he used to drive my eldest brother and

> sometime I used to help him in that as a conductor and sometimes I go to the restaurant I help and sometimes I travel with my dad as well. I study English 5 years I study I think and for writing em anyway in1981 the war started ex-president from Siad Barre? that time of in Somalia. Divided Somalia land is different our restaurant is blow up and my sister was burned with the customer at the same time. I used to play with the ball over there and some of friends kids in Somali in army and say to me your restaurant is blow up and em I was looking for you know my sister and other people already burned and em recognize my sister with gold hair and then I realize they already burned and suddenly my brother comes with the van come on lets go. I say our my sister we have to bury her, he says no we have to go she's gone we cannot do anything.

I wonder what strikes you about this, as material proffered by a research subject to someone (the researcher) with whom he has had no previous relationship? To me, there is a terrible and immediate pain to the narrative which seems strikingly close to the "surface" of the man's mind, not in the least "buried", in fact. And a number of Raelton's interviews have this same quality. The subjects simply dive into the middle of their raw, intensely painful stories, as though these narratives have been lying in wait for someone just willing and able to listen and to be capable of continuing to listen without interruption.

Of course, it is not always like this. Wendy Hollway and Tony Jefferson's (2012) notion of the "defended subject" in narrative research is key, and many subjects are indeed more "defended" than this one. But to me, the brilliance of the method they have elaborated for us is that if as researchers we can bear to allow people to speak, and speak with their whole selves, and if we can have faith in the idea that there is a very great deal "beyond" or "behind" the text or the discourse of the interview, then the project of getting "beneath the surface" is not so difficult. Making sense of what we encounter there is perhaps more difficult, but we will come to that in due course.

This experience—of finding that painful "traumatic narratives" come very directly and immediately to the surface in skilfully conducted narrative interviews—is quite common, and many projects that have engaged professionals in exploration of their everyday experience replicate this feature (Noyes, 2015; O'Sullivan, 2017). "Difficult cases" that have somehow got under the skin of the professional, and psychologically haunt them, sometimes many years after the events concerned, are openly and directly narrated with little prompting. The research interview begins to assume some of the qualities of a therapeutic encounter, with all the attendant ethical questions that arise.

A second level of interpretation

Raelton Gibbs was interested in making sense of how his homeless subjects, carrying with them their exceptionally difficult histories, related to the provision of his organization. He became interested in how all his interviewees seemed, against all the odds, to still be engaged in trying to "make meaning" out of their lives, or in some cases to "find meaning". From this notion, he began to discern the possibility that these people's relationship with, or attachment to, the Salvation Army was significantly about this—if as an organization it was capable of attending to this dimension of its residents' lives and minds. Largely he believes, it is failing to do this, and so the research itself was a quite profoundly troubling process for him, and one that led him gradually into a more critical and questioning stance with respect to his own organization, which incidentally was also sponsoring and paying for his time on the doctoral programme.

There is now something of a leap in the interpretive process, and he generated a diagram to attempt some summative sense of his work (see Figure 14.1). The "leap" is a theoretically informed one, but nonetheless valid for being so. Crucially, the concepts or theory that help to make meaning of the data at this stage must be allowed to "arrive" because the "fit" is good. The data lead the way to the selected theory, not vice versa. In this instance, it was the idea of "hope as a defensive shield" (Potamianou, 1997) that arrived, and Raelton was able to elaborate the concept in relation to his material and link it to other theoretical work about borderline states of mind in clinical and social contexts (Cooper & Lousada, 2005).

His subjects all described what he calls "traumatic histories". Their pathways into both "internal" and external homelessness are intimately bound up with these experiences. A cross-case analysis of their stories, and their states of mind, reveals that they all live on a kind of knife-edge, in a borderline zone, precariously balanced between hope and despair, suicide and survival, life and death, belonging and social inclusion, and isolation and social exclusion (or death). One subject seemed to encapsulate this—he lived part of the time in a hostel, and the rest of his time in a local graveyard. With respect to hope, some subjects seemed to occupy more realistic states of hope and some

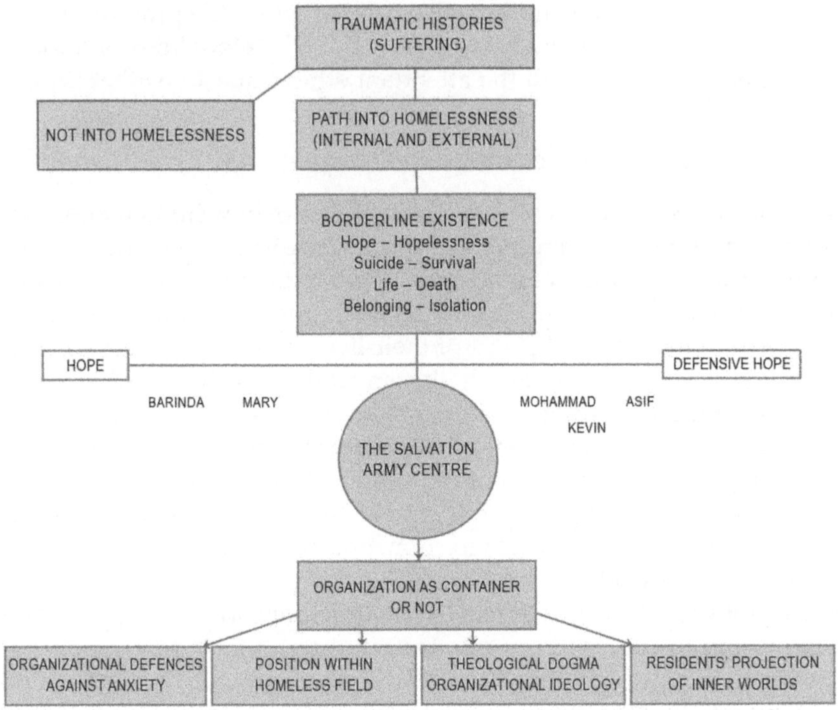

FIGURE 14.1. A pathway to theoretical interpretation. (Courtesy of Raelton Gibbs.)

more defensive ones—an "I know something or someone will arrive to rescue me" state of mind.

So all of this is what they "bring" to the service, the hostel settings in which they live, and in which staff meet and engage, or don't engage, with them. Here you can detect an echo of Bion's famous idea of the container and the contained. Raelton is asking: "What kind of container for these emotional histories, these lives, does the service offer?" Does it engage with them, take them in, offer any space for thinking, digestion of these people's states of mind, or does it defend against such a possibility?

Some premises

I want to attempt to summarize in more abstract form the key premises or assumptions organizing this research programme, which have emerged over the years, and are still emerging.

» First, social workers know from direct experience about particular arenas of social and personal suffering and conflict in our society.

» Second, whether they like it or not, social workers' professional immersion in these social arenas makes of them informal ethnographers of these communities or networks of suffering and conflict. Their "knowledge" is implicitly or explicitly "thickly textured". By virtue of their professional roles, they are also, of course, "positioned" in particular ways in relation to the citizens and groups with whom they work—but, then, so are "researchers" of any description.

» Third, these arenas of private and social experience and relationship in which social workers are typically immersed are characterized by acute and chronic emotional and social pain, and by the anxiety that attends such experiences. These dimensions of social life and experience are typically hidden, marginalized, unreported, and thinly or very intermittently represented in mainstream public discourse.

» Fourth, the capacity to tolerate the mental pain of sustained emotional and professional contact with these realities depends in its turn upon particular psychological and emotional capacities in the practitioner; in turn, the degree of organizational attunement to the needs of practitioners is a key variable in promoting or demoting these capacities.

» Fifth, the capacity to also conceptualize the political and ideological significance of these realities for our society, and for our sense of professional identity, depends on a certain kind of political education that embraces the connection between "private troubles and public issues" (Wright Mills, 1959) and that understands the relationship between private and social suffering.

» Sixth, to undertake meaningful research into these same arenas of private and social experience (whether this focuses primarily on service users' lives or on the practitioner's experience of the work with these populations) requires that similar capacities for depth emotional and political engagement inform the research process itself.

In summary, research rooted in this way of seeing social work and its relationship to both society in general and the experiences of particular individuals, families or groups is crucially dependent on particular psycho-social "capacities of mind". A more developed account of what this means is found in chapters 12 and 15. The theoretical tools associated with these stances are essential, but it is the *capacities of mind, relationship, and emotionally engaged thinking* that are of primary importance, for both practice and research, if we are to enter and return from the underworld with useful knowledge of what happens there.

CHAPTER FIFTEEN

Soft eyes: observation as research

Introduction: the mind as a research instrument

Observation has always been a central strand in our methodologies of discovery, science, social and human inquiry, and all our various attempts to know the world and know ourselves. Some natural sciences such as astronomy are more heavily dependent on observation than others that rely more on experimental testing. However, experimental method also relies heavily on observations in order to test hypotheses and questions. The primary emphasis on observation is also present in certain traditions of social and psychological research such as ethnography and the broad tradition of psycho-social research. However, no one should underestimate either the importance of, or the challenges entailed by, rigorous observation whatever variety of "science" is being pursued. If we have not taken the trouble to thoroughly study what is already there to be "seen", we are at risk of rushing to find explanations and theories for phenomena we cannot even describe fully. Moreover, many answers to important questions are "lying around" if only we know how to look properly. One episode of the famous TV series *The Wire* is called "Soft Eyes" (HBO, 2006). This refers to the police detective discipline of softening the focus of one's vision when searching a crime scene for evidence; the "softer" your eyes, the more likely you are to see the small clue, the unexpected, or the hidden.

Good observational skills are acquired through training and experience, but skill is only part of the story. Observations and the observational method are always theory-laden and context-dependent. It is impossible to make observations free from at least some implicit assumptions, beliefs, theories, or prejudices, although phenomenology—one of the most important traditions in modern social science—began life with just this aim. Observations are always, in the words of one philosopher, "the view from somewhere". The particular tradition of observation which is the concern of this chapter has its own special challenges in this respect, because it relies on the disciplined use of our subjectivity to gather data about the emotional, relational, and unconscious dimensions of other people's subjectivities, relationships, social lives, or organizational milieus. In the words of one valuable writer on this topic, it is about "using the mind as a research instrument" (Skogstad, 2004).

However, the concept of "mind" at work in this chapter is also particular, deriving as it does from applied psychoanalysis. Over the years, a range of psychoanalytic observational methodologies have been developed at the Tavistock Centre, usually as aspects of professional training for mental health workers, psychotherapists, and social workers. These approaches include infant and young child observation, organizational observation, and the observation of "individuals in context". A small but growing tradition of psychoanalytic observational research has subsequently developed as a response to growing confidence in the validity of these methods and their capacity to yield genuine knowledge and understanding of subtle but very influential forces at work in psycho-social life. Postgraduate research students often undertake observations in earlier phases of their professional training, where research is not the main objective, but they come to see the special value of these methods for research as a result. Examples of studies that developed in this way are referred to below.

This chapter discusses briefly how the observational method works and the rules or precepts for conducting safe, rigorous, and productive observations. Then a range of research projects that use psychoanalytic observation are concisely described and reviewed. Following this, some detailed organizational observational material is presented, and then the process by which the observer generated "meaning" from her experience. We then move on to look at some key principles and practices for analysing observational material as research data. Finally, an example is offered of how one researcher integrated several strands of her observational experience to generate a research finding or "formulation".

First, however, it is useful to articulate some broader principles about the nature of psychoanalytic research, of which psychoanalytic observation is just one variety, and to dispel some myths about this way of understanding the world.

What is psychoanalytic research?

Psychoanalytic research uses particular capacities of mind to observe, record, and make sense of unconscious processes in the chosen field of enquiry. The field of enquiry may be a clinical or a therapeutic one, a mainstream social work practice setting involving everyday encounters with clients and colleagues, but equally it may be organizational, community, or policy focused, and so on. But it is the focus on studying unconscious process using clinically derived methods that marks a piece of research out as psychoanalytic, rather than the use of psychoanalytic theory to frame the research project or "make sense" of the data.

This definition assumes that unconscious processes are everywhere, not just in "consulting rooms" or specialized settings in which therapeutic work is happening. The justification for setting out to research a topic in terms of unconscious process will often be framed in terms of "ordinary" professional and social concerns rather than specialized "psychoanalytic" ones—for example, "Can we illuminate the processes via which 'critical incidents' occur and are dealt with in organizations by studying the unconscious dimensions that give rise to them?" Or, "Can psychoanalytic research help us understand the special challenges of everyday child protection work?"

The "capacities of mind" in question are particular—what we might call psychoanalytic clinical capacities—and will usually have been developed and refined through some form of training, namely some or all of: psychoanalytic observational methods, Tavistock work-discussion seminars, psychoanalytic clinical practice, experience of personal psychotherapy, psychoanalytic clinical and/or research supervision, or group relations training.

This formulation positions particular capacities of the researcher at the heart of the research process. The assumption driving this formulation is that unconscious processes within a field of investigation can only be accessed via a researcher who brings his or her emotional and cognitive faculties to bear directly upon that field, via methods of data gathering that facilitate "access to unconscious process". The tried-and-tested practices informing clinical work and observation that enable such access are a central reference point for psychoanalytic research methodology, hence the emphasis noted above on particular training requirements for the practice of psychoanalytic research.

The centrality of the researcher's experiential capacities to the research process means that researcher reflexivity of a particular kind is crucial not just in the process of data gathering, but in data analysis too. Although necessary, the disciplined activity of the trained individual researcher is usually not sufficient to generate the kind of data, and especially the kind of analysis of data, in which we are interested. As we know from clinical practice, at least some of the time the psychoanalytically trained "thinking mind" will need the help of other equally sensitized minds in order to unlock and realize the potential of the material. Thus, the clinical research supervisor or peer-supervision group become, in effect, an extension of or an auxiliary to the psychoanalytic "research mind".

There is something specialized but nothing mysterious about these research capacities and procedures. They can be described, observed, evaluated, and put to work systematically. Eventually, this viewpoint should help locate them as part of a recognized spectrum of qualitative research methods. Most such recognized methods also require training, development, and so on, and some of them also rely on the specialized use of groups to unlock the full potential of the data. Below I expand and develop a number of these themes in relation to observational research.

How does the method work?

The psychoanalytic observational method is characterized by certain precepts that generate the "rules" organizing the method. Many of these principles are shared with other social-scientific observational approaches such as ethnographic observation, but the psychoanalytic focus on emotional experience and unconscious life does require some particular capacities in observers, and some corresponding safeguards against the mental strain that this discipline entails.

First, the observer must negotiate access to the subjects or setting being observed in an open and transparent way. This is for both ethical and methodological reasons. As we shall see, however benign the intentions of the observer may be, the people being observed are inevitably disposed to experience themselves as "under observation". The connotations of this phrase are many and mostly difficult—suicide watch, states of vulnerable physical health, being under suspicion, being stalked, and, most commonly, a fear of being critically examined. Near the end of a twelve-month infant observation I undertook, the baby's older brother toddled over to me and asked "Are you a policeman?" I have known observers who did not negotiate a proper agreement with the observational setting to eventually find they could not tolerate sitting through their hour-long session, so intense was the anxious and questioning gaze that they experienced people being observed turning back upon them, the observer. Also, I have known observers to be refused access, often on seemingly spurious grounds, to organizations such as public libraries and community cafes that permit entry to almost anyone in an unregulated way all the time. The only explanation really is that the prospect of "being observed" arouses too much primitive anxiety.

Second, the observer must be prepared and able to honour his or her "contract" with the observed subjects—for example, to visit the family home to observe a baby for one hour weekly, at an agreed time, for nine months. Again, this is partly about ethics, but it is also about methodology. Observers do affect the situation being observed, and, as we have learned over the years, a part of this impact is that they usually become the object of intense feelings, fantasies, and thoughts. Properly registered, recorded, and understood, these intense experiences turn out to be a gold mine of information about "under-the-surface" or unconscious aspects of the subjectivity, relationships, and organizational struggles of those being observed. In other words, observers mobilize transference relationships in their subjects, and the registration of these in the experience of the observer—the observational countertransference—becomes a key source of new understanding, learning, or, in the case of a research project, data. Put like this, it becomes obvious that one does not break the terms of an observational contract lightly.

Third, the observer must be prepared to tolerate intense, sometimes disturbing, and always to some degree unexpected emotional impacts on themselves arising from the observational experience. So, it is unwise to undertake an observation that is too close to areas of unprocessed mental pain for the observer; the capacity to disentangle which feelings and experiences belong with the observer and which with the observed will be compromised, and too much anxiety on the part of the observer may start to interfere with the "neutrality" that is a key aspect of the observer's role. Psychoanalytic observation is not just a way of learning about "others", but a process of learning about oneself and about the emotional demands of occupying a particular role in which one is required not to intervene or act, except in extremis.

Fourth, the observer needs an appropriate context in which to make sense of his or her material, and undertake the emotional and intellectual "processing" of his or her experience in the service of learning. Usually this takes the form of a weekly, facilitated, small seminar group at which observers make detailed, descriptive presentations of their observational experiences. The seminar group then reflects on and thinks about the meanings embedded in the account. This sustains a focus on the observational task and the learning to be found there and assists in making sense of one's own emotional and cognitive responses as meaningful with respect to the situation being observed. Presenting material in a seminar like this can feel exposing. Sometimes the feelings and thoughts that arise during observations can feel unacceptable, or dangerous, or shameful. But the "fundamental rule" is simple: everything that occurs in the experience of the observer may be relevant, and the task of the seminar is to maintain a non-judgemental and inquiring stance rather than a critical or moralistic one.

Finally, an observer must be prepared for the sometimes arduous task of writing up observations in as much descriptive detail as possible. This is an important discipline in its own right for both clinical learning and for research purposes. It becomes easier with experience, but still it is usually the case that total recall eludes us; often new fragments are suddenly recovered in the course of the day, or night, or during seminar discussions. In psychoanalytic observation, we are in touch with unconscious processes in the observational "field" and, like dreams, these can fade and die, then suddenly revive.

When we deploy psychoanalytic observation in a research project, some or all of the above precepts and "rules" may have to be adapted to the data-gathering circumstances. For example, processing of material may take place in the context of research supervision or seminar groups rather than the reflective observational seminar, and observations may take place in less bounded and controlled circumstances than would be usual in clinical or organizational learning contexts. This is perfectly acceptable, as long as the core ethical and methodological principles outlined above are sustained.

Observation as research

Psychoanalytic observation has been used in a wide variety of research programmes, large and small, both more and less methodologically rigorous and complex, and with greater and less degrees of connection to the "canon" of better established research methodologies. This section briefly reviews some of the most valuable studies and draws out some points of special methodological interest in each of them.

Hinshelwood and Skogstadt's (2000) book is a very good introduction to the method of psychoanalytic observation, and Brown's (2006) paper is a valuable discussion of reflexivity in the observational research process. M. J. Rustin's (1997, 2006) papers provide important philosophical and methodological validation for this variety of observation as legitimate research.

Briggs (1997) undertook six lengthy infant observations in a project that aimed to investigate the fine grain of processes in early development that might differentiate between children who eventually manifest psychological "health" or psychological "risk". He used Grounded Theory (Glaser & Strauss, 2009; Strauss & Corbin, 1998) and declared psychoanalytic conceptual assumptions to analyse his observational data. This study was ground-breaking since it was really the first to deploy observational methods of this variety in a rigorous and systematic way.

Judy Foster (2009, 2016) observed three frontline social work teams with different primary tasks on a total of 45 occasions in her study of "thinking on the front line". Her primary research questions were, "How do social workers think on the front line? What supports their thinking and what gets in the way of it?" and she describes the purpose of the study as "to look at current social work practice and to see how far social workers were able to be creative in helping their clients to 'make a better go of it' given the surface and depth impediments to the task". The notion of "thinking" deployed here is specifically psychoanalytic, stressing the intimate relationship between emotional experiences and our capacity to make sense of, verbalize, and use such experience to inform decision making, assessments, and practice generally, or not, according to the challenges posed by the material requiring "thought". Her methodology combined observations with interviews, and an example of how she analysed her data is given later in this chapter. Her findings included both rich, thickly textured accounts of the different team cultures and the link between these cultures and the teams' primary tasks, and a generalizable typology of what factors assist and what inhibit good team functioning. This project closely informed her later (2016) book *Building Effective Social Work Teams*. As such, the programme of work neatly illustrates how the descriptive, naturalistic study of what "is" can inform a statement of what "can be" in an evidence-based manner.

A recent in-depth evaluation of how a long-established therapeutic community for children actually "works" to produce already well-evidenced outcomes combined psychoanalytic observations of the day-to-day life of the community with interviews, documentary and historical analysis, and some policy contextualization (Price, Herd, Jones, & Sampson, 2017). This project illustrates a key strength of sophisticated observational methodology, namely the capacity to explain the link between psycho-social "mechanisms" that are complex, subtle, non-linear, and which depend on nuanced relationships and interactions, and the effects or outcomes they generate.

Importantly, the staff of the organization under study themselves subscribe to and deploy a psychoanalytic–systems view of their own practice. Thus, their behaviour and thinking with respect to the children resident in the institution is itself "theory-driven" in an explicit way. The theoretical congruence between the organization being studied and the researchers doing the evaluation is perhaps double-edged. Can the researchers really distance themselves sufficiently from those they are studying to be confident they are not simply confirming the "theory of change processes" that the staff of this institution already believe accounts for their success, or impact? On the other hand, could researchers with a limited understanding of the theory of change embedded in the organization's everyday work really achieve an accurate in-depth account of what they were observing? This "double hermeneutic" is not particular to psychoanalytic observation, but reveals the methodological complexities of all psycho-social research endeavours, because all human subjects live their lives on the basis of a range of often implicit rather than explicit theories about their own behaviour.

Hingley-Jones (2008) deployed an adapted form of infant observation with severely learning disabled adolescents and their families with the aim of "bringing together the idea of 'becoming a subject' with the unconscious defensive structures employed by parents in stressful caring situations" (2008, p. 2). Later she comments that

> This form of methodology brings a new perspective to researching severely learning disabled young people as it enables examination of non-verbal, felt and lived experiences which are not adequately

> captured by existing approaches. Although the method incorporates close observation within the family setting, it offers an ethical approach as the observer is required to reflect throughout on how they are influencing the family as well as on how family members are influencing them. [2008, p. 82]

In effect, this study was an early example of the "observation of an individual in context", a method later developed at the Tavistock with the psycho-social concerns of social workers especially in mind. But Hingley-Jones reminds us of another important dimension, or side effect, of skilled observation:

> The opportunity to have an emotionally receptive observer in many cases helped the parents to reflect on their relationships with their learning disabled adolescent and others within the family. This containing function is arguably a forgotten, but vitally important aspect of the professional role which often allowed painful feelings to surface, but sometimes also small movements and change occurred in helpful ways. [pp. 244–245]

Observation may influence the observed participants in helpful and even therapeutic ways.

Hollway's (2015) book *Knowing Mothers* is based on a funded research project to explore identity change in women who are becoming mothers for the first time. Nineteen first time mothers of different ethnicities were engaged in the project. Mothers and their babies were observed weekly for twelve months following the birth, and the women were interviewed three times. Hollway captures well the central strengths of the observational method:

> . . . trained observers become very good at noticing non-verbal, embodied aspects of communication and mental states. The method was therefore consistent with our aim to go beyond the consciously aware, talk-based methods of finding out about identity, wishing to pick up a range of other levels, from the unsaid to the unthinkable; that is those that reside in and are expressed affectively through the body. In other words, our use of psychoanalytically informed observation aimed to go beyond an exclusive methodological focus on text towards a focus on practices and embodied, affective expressions of states of mind and relationship as they are enacted. [2015, p. 47]

This is the most extensive research project to have deployed psychoanalytic observation methods, and it deserves close attention. In some concluding reflections on her own research experience, Hollway also captures some important aspects of the distinctive aims of this variety of research:

> I want to show, not tell; for example, this is what containment looks like in ordinary research encounters, or an example of noticing and following through on a provocation while engaged with data analysis. What is a good balance between showing and theoretical telling is of course uncertain, provisional, and depends on a given specific instance. The pedagogic principle underlying my emphasis on showing through data examples is one further instance of privileging "knowing of". It is based on my intention that readers be able to learn from being affected by the re-told experience on which data analysis is based. Whereas theoretical argument that gets too far removed from the data is liable to feel parched of life . . . [2015, p. 192]

Generating knowledge and understanding

How does observational experience lead to something we can justifiably call knowledge, evidence, or understanding? First, it is important to emphasize that observational study of the kind described above is a variety of empirical inquiry. "Real" phenomena and process are being observed and recorded, both within the observed subjects and within the observer. In other words, feelings, anxieties, wonderings, doubts, spontaneous reveries, and even dreams that seem to be prompted by the observational task are all "facts" of which we can make valid use, as are observations of behaviour, interaction, silences, facial expressions, body language, mood shifts, and so on.

The meaning, interpretation, or status of what is observed and recorded when we attend to all these dimensions of a situation may indeed be very "slippery", uncertain, open to various lines of interpretation, and likely to remain contested, but in itself this is no barrier to the effort to achieve a "formulation" of what we think is occurring in the situations observed. Indeed, it is because ordinary as well as unusual human psychological and social processes are complex and multi-layered that we need subtle and perhaps unfamiliar "ways of knowing" in order to grasp them better. The subtler epistemological questions associated with observation as a research method are more fully explored in Price and Cooper (2012).

A complex boundary crossing

In the illustration that follows we can notice a number of the ideas outlined above as they unfold in the experiences and then the written reflective analysis of one observer, Nicola O'Sullivan.[1] She has chosen to undertake a ten-week organizational observation in a sexual health centre in the city where she works. As she realizes later, this "choice" may not have been very "conscious" on her part, and this in itself generates a combination of unexpected anxiety in her but also deep learning and personal reflection. There are early signs of what is to come in the opening paragraph of her first observational record, in which she is to meet the Director of the centre and the staff:

> Usually when I leave for appointments I let the staff team know where I am going and the purpose of my visit there. This morning, during the handover, I alerted the staff team on duty as to my plans for the day. I had appointments with a social work team, meeting a parent in the afternoon to review her placement and then said that I was heading to the sexual health clinic for 10.30 am. There was silence in the room. I too felt something, perhaps unease or embarrassment, I am not sure. I continued to chat about other things, with the unease sitting in the air in the office.

By the time she has parked, she is late.

> I continued to search the side streets for the place. I considered how closely my trying to get there was connected to other women and men who for whatever reasons have to make the journey to this centre for support with their sexual health needs. I thought about my own sexual health needs, my age and my relationship.
>
> On arrival I sat on the seat nearest to the door; I noticed an engraving on the window of the front door of a sperm. I noticed then a fish tank in front of me to the right of a table of magazines. Cameron Diaz was on the front of one of the magazines, I thought about what it must be like to be her. I then watched the fish, they were beautiful, tiny, luminous fish, swimming in the tank, but with no direction it seemed to me.

In retrospect, of course, the observer wonders why she allowed herself to be late for this appointment. But already, as she notices and later records the stream of her own thoughts, some possible answers to this question take shape. She is thinking about "my own sexual health needs, my age, my relationship". Suddenly, as long as she can capture and retain this experience, she may have some insight into what it is like to be a user of this service, and what states of anxiety and trepidation are carried across the organizational boundary into the reception area, where she will soon decide to position herself for her observational sessions.

Despite her state of heightened anxiety, or perhaps partly because of it, she is very alert to the signs and symbols that present themselves as she enters the physical but also the experiential field of the organization. An engraving of a sperm (can it really be so, and why a sperm, not an egg, or something else?), a magazine with a picture of a female celebrity, and a tank with tiny, luminous fish swimming "but with no direction it seemed to me". Now, these tiny fish are innocent participants in the scene, and if, as I think we are intended to understand, they also suggest to the observer an idea of sperm swimming in semen, then this fragment of "meaning" is both entirely her own but also a meaning that might plausibly be evoked for others, given the context in which they are seen. Perhaps you, the reader, had the same thought, or one could certainly imagine more than one member of a seminar group doing so. The observer, alive to the moment-by-moment flow of her *own subjective experience of the organizational setting*, has entered what I have called the "dream space" of the observation, a somewhat disorderly but perhaps meaningful domain of symbols, associations, feelings, and thoughts (see chapter 14).

The observer is met by the receptionist and taken to meet Deirdre, the Director.

> The Director introduced me to Madeleine, it seemed she was her right-hand woman although I wasn't sure. Madeleine shook my hand and I apologized again for being late. I was trying to manage the tension in the air, which might have been both my own and their nervousness at this new adventure we were both embarking on.

There is some quite lengthy preliminary discussion about the purpose of the observation.

> I listened and then I gave them the letter from the Tavistock explaining the process of organizational observation. The Director asked for further explanation. I suggested that over the ten weeks I would come to the centre and spend the hour in the reception area. Both she and Madeleine spent some time talking to me about how boring it would be in the reception area. Deirdre explained that I wouldn't see anything or any young people particularly on a Wednesday. They thought I would get much more from visiting schools.

At this point the observer has to hold her ground, which she manages successfully.

> Then the Director asked if I knew what had happened to their team last year. She told me that a member of an anti-abortion organization had come in to use their service and presented falsely as a client and had tried to encourage one of their counsellors to break the law, they had videotaped the whole counselling session and supplied the video tapes to a national editor of a newspaper, also a pro-life campaigner.

This observer has only just "negotiated entry" to the organization, but already rather a lot has happened! It seems the observer's anxiety about presenting herself for the first time may have led her to be late. In her first encounters with the Director and her colleague, we see her apologizing twice, and clearly she is rather flustered. Here the "action" of the observer's anxiety is intruding somewhat on her capacity to manage herself in role as a prospective observer. Never mind—all we can do is learn from such experiences, and use this learning to once again think about what states of mind staff in this setting are probably routinely faced with as their clients "cross the boundary" of the centre, carrying their conflicts and anxieties with them. Importantly, the observer has a real *experience* of such a state of mind, and this is a simple example of the "depth understanding" of organizational processes that observation can deliver.

Next, it transpires that there are rather unusual "reality" factors informing the organization's state of mind as they receive the observer for the first time. We noted above that observers can readily elicit fears in those they are observing about being under hostile scrutiny. But in this case, the organization has actually been the object of a covert, hostile, and deceitful attempt to attack their work. Some organizations are more likely than others to be anxious about such possibilities. External anxiety-inducing reality factors mingle with less conscious "internal" anxieties and together produce a complex psycho-social reality. Importantly, however, very similar organizations are found to handle these anxieties very differently, and the same is true of private households. For example, how trusting or suspicious or anxious is the organizational or family culture—or, indeed, the infant or adult being observed—with respect to the "outside world"? In the case we are looking at, it seems that there may be quite a high degree of basic trust, despite the experiences they have had.

In sum, it may be that a combination of the observer's capacity to manage her own anxiety well enough, the help afforded by the letter she presents which acts as some kind of "warrant", and the organization's own capacity for basic trust combine to facilitate her successful entry. Phew.

Meaning takes shape: contamination anxieties

Over ten weeks, the observer presents herself for her hourly session in the reception area of the Centre, and gradually a set of difficult meanings emerge. The experience becomes something of a test of endurance. Later she writes that

> From the moment I walked toward the Centre I was "allergic" and this feeling of being allergic was to re-emerge at each and every visit and was to form my experience of projective identification and countertransference.

In the reception area she observes, she is subjected to a variety of experiences associated with this allergic feeling.

> I realized that the space which was the reception area also acted as in some way the "treatment" space for the staff team and clients. Here their defensive strategies against the threatening emotions of what their task held up for them were played out. This was clearly experienced in the emotions and behaviours manifested in the process of cleaning the reception area. This was a weekly event which caused me considerable distress and anxiety experienced in the countertransference; on a surface level this cleaning took on a humorous aspect and I was at times animated in my recalling of this experience in my seminar group.
>
> The receptionist had now begun cleaning the reception table, I thought was this because of me or was it a Wednesday morning ritual. The receptionist continued cleaning tables in the reception area while the other gentleman continued hovering . . . a young man and woman came in, the receptionist joked with them . . . he continued cleaning, he began to clean outside the building now, the window behind my head.
>
> I felt overwhelmingly that whatever was in the reception area, including me, had to be cleaned or might contaminate it. These feelings were perhaps reflective of the organization's feelings of disgust or disdain for

> their clients, but could not be openly spoken about so were managed in this way and in the smiling and offering of tea and coffee. I wondered about the space for open holding and managing of anxiety.
>
> There is a lot of rummaging behind the wall of reception, the receptionist returns with another counsellor I think and a hoover, I discover this is a steam cleaner. I think about the cleaning and then a strong smell of lavender spray hits me almost between my eyes, the receptionist has begun spraying the reception area ... the steamer is on, they clean vigorously as they sing, I am anxious as the steamer approaches me, I have to lift my legs while I am almost washed away.

And so the observer is able to achieve an initial "formulation" about the psycho-social anxieties that inform the organization's functioning at a level that is in one sense "under the surface" but in another was there for anyone to notice if they attend to their experience in the right way.

> The emotional experience of this organization was felt in this instance at a physical level and emerged in their incessant cleaning. The climate of repression in matters sexual shaped the imagery and language within which relationships and sex were experienced in the national culture. Sex was associated explicitly and implicitly with feelings of shame, guilt and embarrassment. The emotional significance of what this organization or its members were doing is bound up in the systems and culture and is being held in the confined space of the reception area, without explanation, or attention.

In the final section of this chapter, we see how a formulation about the connection between an organization's task, the anxieties inherent in its work processes, and a researcher's observational records of her experiences are handled in a systematic and methodologically rigorous manner to arrive at a research "finding".

Analysing observational data

The process of making sense or meaning from the observations occurs partly through attendance at regular seminars or supervisions, but importantly also through the act of "writing up" the whole experience in a summative manner. But when observation is used as part of a research project, the requirements of research methodology and more systematic strategies for data analysis enter the picture. In the end, the kind of meaning-oriented formulation described above is always what we are aiming for, but the route towards it must be systematic, rigorous, transparent, and open to independent checks.

There is no "off-the-shelf" method for analysing observational data, nor does this section aim to be a "manual" for undertaking this task. Here I suggest that an approach to analysing data that incorporates the following elements is helpful:

» A respect for many of the principles of classic ethnographic research. Ethnography is a part of the social-scientific methodological canon and, like psychoanalytic observation, is a form of "naturalistic inquiry" involving immersion in social or psycho-social situations.
» An approach that integrates inductive ("bottom-up") and deductive ("top-down") strategies, which also keep the whole field of the observation in mind while paying close attention to the parts, the particulars, and the fine detail. The notion of fluid movement back and forth between "figure and ground" from Gestalt theory is useful in this respect (see Hollway & Jefferson, 2012). Strategies that overemphasize inductive procedures risk losing sight of the bigger picture, while those that lay too much weight on deduction risk failing to engage with the elements of data that may surprise, puzzle us, or challenge and question the observer's assumptions and settled beliefs.
» Disciplined recording and then analysis of the observer's emotional experience of the observations, as well as the record of "what happened". This process should enable the researcher to identify genuine countertransference experiences, which are a rich source of data for the eventual process of "making meaning".
» The use of a research seminar or group to supplement and support the researcher's individual data-analytic efforts. The importance and value of having several trained minds going to work (even just a couple of times) on psychoanalytically informed data is discussed more fully in Price and Cooper (2012) and in chapter 14.

Ethnographic principles

One can do ethnography without undertaking psychoanalytic observation, and, likewise, we can use observation as a research method without becoming a full-blown ethnographer. But the inherent link between the two approaches is that they are "naturalistic" methods that entail immersion in other people's lived experience. Among studies cited in this chapter, Foster's (2009, 2016) work and Price et al.'s (2017) study probably most closely approach classic ethnography.

Hammersley (1992) proposes that readers of good ethnography should have ways of being able to judge the validity and relevance of the research, especially the validity of truth claims made, on the basis of the adequacy of the evidence offered in support of them. These are useful principles to bear in mind when assessing the merits of one's own or others' observational research. For a fuller account of these principles, see Hammersley (1992), p. 64.

Inductive and deductive strategies

Many qualitative methodologies emphasize the need to break down textual research data into small individual units, followed by a search for links between these units to create initial "codes" or themes, which are then subject to a further search for links and patterns. These second-order "codes" may then suggest new ways of searching for patterns in the lower levels of raw data. Second-order codes may also be drawn together into families that begin to suggest the presence of a concept or overarching theme present in the data. Again, there may be a return to the lower levels of data to see if these are now differently illuminated. This process of "iteration" is arduous and time consuming, but it is fundamental to the "inductive method"—working from an assembly of particulars in the direction of a generalization or formulation that captures something more than just the sum of the parts. But how do we justify this leap "beyond the particulars", the jump to "something more than just the sum of the parts"?

This is the problem of the inductive method: classical logic suggests that there is no way to validly infer a generalization or universal from a series of particulars. Because the sun rose this morning, and yesterday, and the day before—indeed appears to have done so since the beginning of time—we are not actually *logically* justified in predicting that it will do so tomorrow, and simply piling up more and more observations of the same behaviour does not get you any closer to solving the problem. No amount of repeated observations can get us to a statement of a "law"—"The sun always rises".

I propose the following steps as a guide to the process of moving from raw data elements to a meaningful interpretation:

1. We notice some "patterns" (something similar to an instance of "law-like" regularity) in the data that seem consistent. For

example, in the observation described above, the observer finds herself *repeatedly* a witness to or a subject of efforts to "clean her away". She is entitled to link these separate observations, and make something of them.

2. At the simplest level, we can just give a name to this apparent patterning or consistency in the data and perhaps notice its similarity to other patterns or generalizations we know of from the literature. In our example, the notion of "contamination anxiety" is somewhat original, and that in itself is an achievement.
3. But a stronger approach is to locate a theoretical or conceptual framework that "fits", or illuminates or *interprets*, the data and renders them "meaningful" within a wider context. Because the data we are interested in were genuinely discovered, this theoretical step may move us beyond any hypotheses or hunches inscribed in the research questions that drove the project at the outset. It is a *discovery* that this theoretical formulation might be applicable to *this* data, and if this is convincing, it may extend or modify the original theoretical formulation in interesting ways. The blend of new and original data illuminated by more familiar concepts or theory allows us to capture *both* the uniqueness of the situation we have observed, *and* its relationship to other already better known, similar "cases", or to a context that seems to fit. In our example, the observer proposes that a history of cultural repression and anxiety about sex is condensed inside the work of the agency, complicating its primary task in conflictual and anxiety-laden ways. It would be interesting to observe a similar centre in another part of the same country, or another society, and compare the findings. Briggs's (1997) study also exemplifies this approach when he locates a resonance between his own findings and a prior theoretical schema of different types of containment, or lack of it, between infant and carer. In this way, we contribute to the project of "theory building" or "theory extension". Our map of "reality" is just a bit richer and deeper, but in an evidenced way.

Some contemporary methodologists engage with the problems of inductivism and deductivism by drawing on the work of, first, C. S. Peirce who proposed a third logical principle—retroduction or abduction—and, second, the more recent school of critical realist philosophers who have developed systematic theoretical models for dealing with the "gap" between inductive strategies and deductive ones. The moment of theorization, or hypothesis formulation, that introduces conceptual order into a series of observationally based inductive findings is the first step in a "retroductive" strategy. It is called retroduction because having postulated a hypothesis to "explain" or account for the patterns in the data, one is then obliged to test the hypothesis (in a more deductive manner) by returning to examine and test further the empirical observations or hypotheses that first generated the explanation. For a fuller accessible account of all of this see Blaikie (1993).

Recording and access to countertransference data

When we write up observational experiences, it is important to capture as much of what occurred in the hour-long session as possible, both externally in terms of behaviours, conversation, and silences and also "internally" in terms of the observer's feelings, thoughts, sense of emotional atmospheres, and bodily responses. But equally important is to stay descriptive at this stage and to avoid premature interpretation or theorization. This discipline allows for a more open and inquiring approach to the question, "What might be happening at an unconscious level in this observation?" (A good discussion of the methodological issues associated with the discipline of recording and of the epistemological status of such textual records is given in chapter 4 of Price, 2004, who undertook detailed observations of primary-school children and their teachers.)

The question of what exactly the unconscious "is", or how it can be noticed and made sense of in observational work, is too broad to venture into in depth in this chapter. I like to work with the following fairly simple ideas. First, I assume that unconscious processes are everywhere, not just in "consulting rooms" or specialized settings in which therapeutic work is happening. This is consistent with those psychoanalytic thinkers who also work with the idea of a "field" and with Ogden's formulation, as noted in chapter 14, about the nature and location of the unconscious:

> The unconscious is not "subconscious"; it is an aspect of the indivisible totality of consciousness. Similarly meaning (including unconscious meaning) is *in* the language being used, not under or behind it. (Freud [1915e] believed the term "subconscious" to be "incorrect and misleading" since the Unconscious does not lie "under" consciousness.) [Ogden, 1999, p. 215]

The challenge that immediately arises from the notion of the observer as part of an unconscious field of experience is how to establish what elements of the total experience "belong" to the observational setting, and what to the observer. I want to suggest that in both the example offered above and in the final section of this chapter, we see this process of sense-making at work involving both the external "realities" and the more private responses of observers; disentangling these is important, but not so that one can be privileged over another—both make equally relevant contributions to the generation of meaning in the observation.

The central message here is that "the unconscious" is not such a difficult and mysterious phenomenon to capture if one can be sufficiently open to one's own emotional experience within the total "field" of the observation.

Using a supervision group

However, as discussed towards the opening of this chapter, it remains true that we often do need help with the process of seeing and making sense of what is "lying about" in the psycho-social world. Clinical experience shows us that the best-trained psychoanalytic practitioners need the help of other equally sensitized minds in order to unlock and realize the potential of the material. The research supervisor or peer-supervision group become, in effect, an auxiliary to the psychoanalytic "research mind". Figure 15.1 tries to represent the process of translating unconscious processes captured in the data into legible, usable data elements. The model is indebted to Bion's thinking about the process of reverie and the role of containment in enabling thoughts that take shape as "beta elements" become transformed with the aid of what he termed "alpha function", as they are "won from the formless void and infinite", which is the realm of the unconscious.

Transference, countertransference, unconscious identifications, and projection of unprocessed material into the research supervision arena are not a problem, but are the richest and most valuable means of accessing the unconscious dimensions of the field of inquiry.

Reaching a formulation: one social work team's culture and anxieties

In the extract below from Judy Foster's study of how front-line social work team's "think" and work in relation to their tasks, she links various levels of data under the broad heading of "countertransference" in search of a formulation that captures something about the connections between her own experience as an observer, the culture

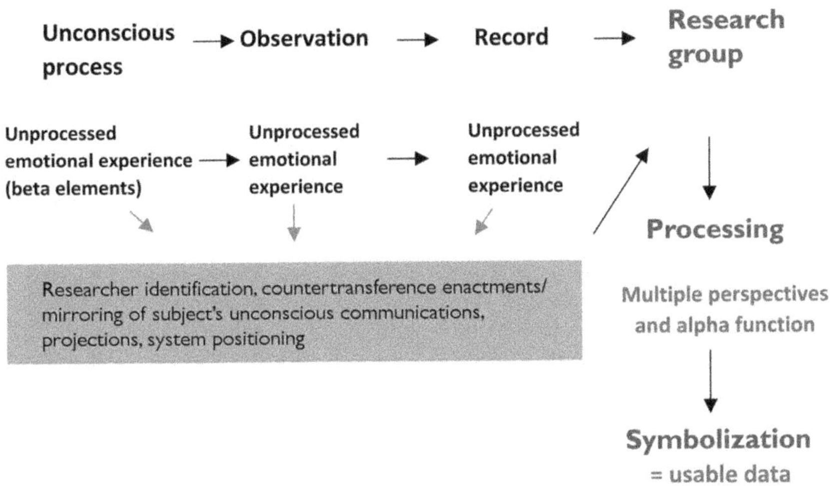

FIGURE 15.1. The role of the research supervision group in psychoanalytic observational research.

and atmosphere of team dynamics and functioning, and the task they have as a team. The elements she combines include:

1. Recognition of the specific anxieties the team have about the "damaging" impact they feel they may have on their clients. These are linked to the specificity of the "objective" task of "having to act in a punitive way" for the clients' long-term benefit.
2. Her own "reverie" about a situation at home in which she had felt "damaging".
3. The power of the team's transference to her as an intrusive, inspectorial figure, who records their interactions and "makes them paranoid".
4. Her inability to sustain her observational role in the face of their persecutory feelings about her.
5. Her "enactment" in leaving her notebook at the observation site—the only occasion on which she did this across numerous observations in three teams.
6. The apposite force of a stray comment by a friend—"Have you finished your surveillance yet?"
7. Theoretical references that help to "make sense" of the total experience.

My first observation visit was to the Monday team meeting. The team were discussing applications for a hostel vacancy, where one of the applicants was said to be violent and unpredictable. I found myself in an unpleasant reverie. Rather than listening to the discussion, I was preoccupied with a difficult situation at home which had left me feeling damaging and incompetent. This stray thought of mine (Ogden, 1999) may have been a counter-transference experience to give insight into one of the group's concerns. As I learnt more about the team's work I realised that they often felt damaging when trying to help their clients. They were preoccupied with the dilemma of having to act in a punitive way for the client's long term good.

At the end of Visit 6 I forgot my notebook. It was left amongst some papers on the spare desk. On my return I found an unsigned note slipped between the pages "Please do not leave this around, it makes us feel paranoid". My forgetting the notebook and their reaction to it illustrated the strong persecutory dynamic in observing and being observed.

I endured several uncomfortable sessions of which my final piece of observation was typical:

> *At this point (about half an hour into the meeting) there was some complex banter and sharp remarks (I think Ed said something OTT about another member of staff)—people looked at me to see my reaction—was I writing it down? I felt very intrusive and uncomfortable and deliberately put down my pen for a bit. Twenty minutes later the quick talk became quicker and Ed made a sharp in joke about Fraser that I missed. Everyone looked at me to see how I'd reacted. I said—"I missed that" and put down my pen and stopped writing. The meeting came to an end. I mentioned that it was the end of Part One of my research and there would no more observation (Visit 9M).*

The group eventually pressured me to stop making notes. I felt compelled to put my pen down, unable to continue recording due to the intensity of feeling in the group. The group used Ed's sharp tongue to attack me as the outsider, just as they used him to express their frustration with their clients and each other. I could not continue. I told them that this was my last piece of observation. That evening a friend asked me "Have you finished your surveillance yet?" precisely articulating [this group's] emotions.

What was all this about? Admittedly being observed is never comfortable. Healy (1998) points out "Being observed, especially if we are being observed in a crisis situation, may evoke the feeling of dread that what we are doing is wrong and will be exposed to the world for critical judgement." And again on audit, "Superego type audit activity is characterised by a dread or terror in those being audited of being found out, being criticised and being harshly judged" (pp. 54–55). But the Mental Health Team were working with a particular group of service users who were more than homeless. Gilligan (1996, cited in Adlam & Scanlon, 2005) suggests that "such people are made to feel ashamed, not only of what they do, but the deeper wounding of being ashamed of who they are: literally ashamed of their self" (p. 457). Steiner (2006) reminds us that "humiliation is an important part of the threat coming from superego figures" (p. 941). Observation had therefore a particular emotional meaning for the Mental Health Team which was managed sensitively for their clients. I had no such dispensation and felt the full force of their projections. [Foster, 2009, p. 132]

Conclusion

This chapter has attempted to provide a reasonably in-depth introduction to the practice and theory of psychoanalytic observation as a research method. There is much more that could be discussed, and the interested reader is encouraged to pursue some of the references within the chapter. The examples and illustrations have also drawn heavily on organizational and psycho-social material rather than infant or young-child observation. The key research challenges and debates are slightly different according to the object of study, but again the reader can pursue their particular interests through further reading. However, in the end there is only one way to learn about this or any other research method—go and try it, and learn from experience.

Note

1. The case material in this section is from an unpublished professional doctorate assignment on "Organizational Observation" written by Nicola O'Sullivan in 2013 for the Tavistock Centre/University of East London (available from: acooper@tavi-port.nhs.uk).

PART V

AND FINALLY . . .

CHAPTER SIXTEEN

Hearing the bluebird sing: on death, dying, and social work

Meaning, containment, and communication

In December 2016, Margot Waddell presented a paper at the monthly Tavistock Scientific Meeting entitled "'And so of larger— Darknesses—' Living with Dying: The Containing Function of Meaning". Her delivery of the paper generated a unique atmosphere among the packed audience, and the chair commented towards the end of the discussion that he had never before experienced the particular quality of silence that took hold of the room at points, in the spaces between contributions from the floor. My own thought was that this atmosphere was produced by the degree and intensity of emotional work that Margot had undertaken with respect to her theme over a period of about eighteen months following a first version of the paper she delivered at a conference on the subject of "Living with Dying". To me, her 2016 presentation was a rare phenomenon, in which she generated a "lived experience" of psychoanalysis for, and within, a live audience.

What exactly does this mean? The paper concerned the way in which art—poetry and novels especially, in the examples she used—can engage with deep anxieties and other troubling or unthinkable realms of experience and render them communicable and thinkable by giving them symbolic form, which is to say "meaning". This in turn is very close to what Bion intended to connote by the expression "containment". Arguably, the whole aim of psychoanalytic work of any kind is captured in such a formulation: the extension or deepening of our capacity to tolerate thinking thoughts we would rather not think, and to feel the feelings associated with such thoughts. An effective psychoanalytic "interpretation" achieves just this, by catching, holding, and giving symbolic form to a slippery (because unwelcome) experience we already carry within ourselves. Such a moment is marked by both emotional relief and cognitive recognition, an experience of "insight". Importantly, I think this process is always relational, one in which another mind, or a thinking part of our own mind, comes to the aid of a part of us that is struggling to make sense of emotional experience. The reciprocal process of conveying understanding to another, and of being understood, becomes an encounter with truth, specifically emotional truth.

These observations return me to the opening paragraphs of the introduction to this book, in which I wrote about "writing differently", an experience of being led from within by a search for meaning in the act of writing, rather than just from without in a search for intellectual coherence, or, perhaps, academic recognition. I do not seek any comparison between the quality of writing or depth of working through in the present chapter, or any other in this book, and what Margot Waddell achieved in her communication that day, but the aspiration is perhaps the same: to bring something alive for readers, as much as to transmit knowledge.

In writing about death and dying, it is difficult to avoid the cliché that "we are all mortal" and that this might be what is "unthinkable" for each of us. In this chapter, I hope not to evade that truth; primarily I want to engage readers in a slightly different exploration, which is with experiences of "death in our lives". For we all have these inside us, even if we might superficially believe that, fortunately, no one really close to us has yet died and we have been thus far spared. I approach this project through reflections on experiences of death and dying in my own life, and a tentative exploration of the connections between these and my career choices as a social worker and psychotherapist.

As a society, it seems we are more and more interested in death and dying, while we still recognize death as one of the so-called last taboos. Most weeks *The Guardian* carries at least one piece about dying, including quite frequent reviews of the memoirs of dying people, or of the dying of a loved one. Even as I was drafting this talk, I noticed and read a long, difficult but courageous piece by a doctor, "How Do People Die from Cancer?" (Srivastava, 2016), and another about how gardening is not really about life and nurture but death and destruction. Some people systematically research death and dying, some write about their professional experiences of working in the hospice and palliative-care system or child-bereavement counselling services, others write their memoirs, and poets and novelists have always written about death. My method, if it can be called that, is slightly different again. I am alive and pretty well, all things considered. But I feel death has stalked me for much of my life, and a few years ago I began to write about the presence of death in my life. A nasty bout of pneumonia that took some weeks to resolve seemed to be the prompt for this. I felt horribly unwell, and I know I was afraid, rationally or not, that I might be dying. The experience revived deep-seated memories, carried as much in my body as my mind, I suspect, of much earlier serious illnesses in my life and more definite encounters I had had with the possibility of death.

Nothing to fear but fear itself

Perhaps such experiences reveal that fears about dying lie just under the surface of our awareness all the time. Illness, loss, and transitions of many kinds may bring us into temporary, closer contact with death anxiety. This is a thought to which I return later, because just possibly it discloses something fundamental about the deeper meaning of social work as an activity and as a wider social purpose. To be aware of our mortality all the time would be impossible, a state of permanent terror. And yet I think this is exactly what we encounter in many of the traumatized children, young people, and adults with whom we work. Rarely will it present transparently or legibly, but the emotional and relational intensity of what we may call, among many possibilities, attachment disorders, suicidality, or serious self-harm usually has roots in a terror of abandonment and separation that is, at bottom, a fear of dying in the absence of the protective presence of another person. When we as professionals step into the scene, this intensity can be readily transferred onto us. Fear of dying may be so intense that it communicates itself as an effort to kill the other person—us—or it may be so intolerable that actual death comes to seem preferable to going on living in a state of continual terror.

I once remarked to a psychotherapy patient that it seemed she had never suffered a significant bereavement. She was in her early forties by now. She had endured very real childhood emotional struggles and deprivations, but I sensed that somehow nothing had ever really shaken her, and so she tended to stay stuck with her misery. Death in our lives changes us irrevocably, but I think never in ways we can anticipate. Paradoxically, perhaps, I felt this woman could not yet live properly because she had not really encountered death.

More often than we realize, I suspect, we are inhabited by the struggles with dying and death endured by our parents and by their parents in turn, and so on. Such experiences of death and dying live on within us. In this country, all except the oldest generations know very little directly of the horrors of war. But war, and the psychological after-burdens of war, live on in us, and our relation to the wars being conducted at the thresholds of our society now are part of my concern in this chapter.

Stalking the stalker: the primitive edge of experience

In her memoir of the process of her own dying, *Late Fragments,* Kate Gross (2015) describes an experience of vivid mental and emotional lucidity in the face of her terminal diagnosis. The book is written to, and for, her two very young and soon-to-be-motherless children. But its emotional urgency seems to have other sources as well, an effort to meet death and come to know it—track it down, maybe—as best she could, as a way of securing for herself and others the meaning of her life. I stopped feeling impelled to write about death once my illness remitted; from time to time I have picked it up again, only then to lose—not interest—but my ability to engage with the project. Like Kate Gross, fragments are all I manage to produce. The mental and emotional strain of thinking about dying is immense, and it propels us towards a primitive edge of our experience. When I was reading Kate Gross's book, a particular passage prompted the train of thought about my patient who had not encountered dying, and more ideas as well. A few seconds later I could recall nothing of what I had been thinking, like a dream remembered and then forgotten. It took a strenuous conscious effort of will to recover the thoughts from the void to which they had returned. So I think it is ordinary to find we can sustain emotional contact with "thinking about dying" for only so long before we retreat or turn away. We can stalk our own relation to dying and death but never finally capture it.

Strange meeting

I lived in the same house for the first nine years of my life, a large rectory on a hill outside a Bedfordshire village. Forty years later, I took my wife to see it, and to visit my parents' graves in the nearby churchyard. We walked up the long driveway. The front door of the house was ajar, and my wife encouraged me to knock. A woman came, and I said, "My name is Andrew Cooper, and I used to live here." She looked at me for a moment and said, "Of course you did, come in." It was as though time had telescoped, the decades had not elapsed, and she had always been expecting me. When my family moved, she and her husband and their five young children had bought the house. A year later, her husband died of cancer. She recounted how, in one of their last conversations, he said, "Don't sell the house." Her children were now grown up with families of their own, and one of her sons now owned a nearby farm. She pointed to the hillside opposite where a tractor and plough were moving slowly across the horizon. "There he is", she said.

The house had hardly changed. There had been no money. The cream "pebbled" wallpaper I remembered from childhood still lined the dining-room walls. It was a large place by any standards, with a walled garden, a garage that had once been stables, and a "billiard room". Here she showed us an old-fashioned coal-fired boiler and told how one night, alone in the house with the children, she had heard a terrible bang, like a clap of thunder. The boiler had exploded in some way, and it had never been used since. The story of the night it exploded seemed to stand for the catastrophe of death, and the object itself for the husk of a past life, a memorial standing in a room that, one sensed, she rarely entered, around which life had continued.

The whole experience had a dream-like quality in which past, present, and future were condensed and indistinguishable. There is something of this in most of the stories I have to tell. I think close contact with experiences of death and dying involves entry into a realm of timelessness, where something is frozen.

Becoming a social worker

In deeper layers of the mind, I suspect all separations or endings are experienced as deaths or portents of death. After we left my childhood home and moved to another large, draughty rectory, I was deeply distressed, but not in ways that felt communicable. So I behaved strangely, in ways that perturbed my parents and perplexed others. The move coincided with other transitions in the family. My much older twin brothers left to go to university. My even older eldest brother married and moved into the new family home with his wife. She was not whom my parents would have wished for their first-born son. The newly-wed couple argued, and the wife wept. Then she became pregnant. Upstairs my mother wept uncontrollably, perhaps because she had been happy in the village we had left, because her children were growing away, perhaps because she was menopausal as well—another kind of death that all women must traverse. The new house was filled with anxiety and a sense of my father's, and everyone's, helplessness. The ten years my family lived in the rectory on the hill passed into our family mythology as a kind of lost golden age.

I am narrating these memories in part because I believe they suggest something about my eventual choice of career as a social worker. I was the son of a parish priest, and my mother played an equally vital role for the communities they ministered to with her tireless work organizing pastoral care—young mothers groups, coffee mornings, Women's Institute work, keep-fit classes, and less tangibly just her formidable and endless attention to sustaining relationships. She was very good at this work but also, I think, deeply frustrated to have abandoned a professional career of her own, for which she was qualified and absolutely capable. The family atmosphere and culture was not easy for me. Conflicts and distress were not openly or comfortably handled or processed. As by far the youngest member of the family, isolated from ordinary village life and connections, I absorbed the abundant anxieties and tensions without knowing I was doing so. In my twenties, following my father's death after a lengthy dementia, sibling tensions among my brothers erupted, and there was a protracted rupture between my oldest brother's family and my mother. But I steered clear of taking sides, and for some period of time in my twenties I was the only family member on speaking terms with everyone else.

Someone once said that a psychotherapist is a person who has not given up hope of curing their parents. For myself, I think I chose social work as a way of continuing to try to heal my whole family and, beyond this, to continue my parents' work of healing and sustaining communities. Church-going and the demands of religious practice and ritual simply bored me as a child, and consciously I rejected any identification with Christianity. However, by the time I was a qualified social worker in a patch-based community team in Earls Court, I had come to recognize, or believe, that I was, in a secular form, "about my father's business",[1] and also my mother's. One of my more successful efforts as a patch social worker was to organize an Over-50's Health Club for local residents, which met in a local church hall. But it was mental health work that engaged me most deeply, and eventually I did train as a psychotherapist too.

Grief interrupted

Death and dying are transgenerational processes. How the generations that preceded us handled them profoundly affects each of us. Whether or not we have been able to modify and transform this impact has equally weighty consequences for ourselves and then for our children, and so on. My mother was an only child, and my father's only sibling, his brother Oliver, was killed in the First World War. My eldest brother's middle name was also Oliver, and this was the name by which he was always known. A striking sepia photographic portrait of our long-dead uncle—a beautiful young man, a boy really, in his Scottish regimental uniform—hung in every house in which we lived. My mother often remarked to me that I strongly resembled him, though I find the likeness hard to see. So probably it was the link she forged between us that so sensitized me to the stories she told of him, and not any connection I made for myself. Still, when my mother died, I urgently claimed this portrait in the division of family heirlooms. It felt like a part of me. To this day, I struggle to recount the following story, often narrated to me by my mother, without crying.

In his youth, my father was a member of the Boys Brigade in Glasgow. He played the bugle and was to perform the "Last Post" at the ceremony immediately following the arrival of the news of his brother's death in Greece. His best friend stood by with his own bugle in case my father fainted, ready to pick up the melody wherever my father left off. He did faint but, according to my mother, no one noticed so smoothly did his friend segue with his own playing.

But did it really happen like this? Or was the story itself somehow smoothed over, polished up by my mother to hone its emotional or perhaps sentimentalizing impact? The tale seems to speak of unthinkable grief that is not allowed to disrupt the surface of the ritual that marks it. And the story carries a suggestion of cruelty, or mindlessness: how could a boy of 14 be expected to play the "Last Post" at such a time? Or is this just a reminder to us of military discipline, of what people endure in terms of holding on to grief when circumstances require that they "keep calm and carry on"? Is this why it still affects me so, because the awful fragmenting power of my father's loss never was released to do the destructive but also reparative emotional work that true mourning must contend with? I do not know. I know only that these events, or rather their narrations, were smuggled into my mind where they still search for articulation, for meaning. At one time in my life I would sit alone and read the poems of Wilfred Owen, hardly more than a boy himself when he was killed a few days before the 1918 armistice, and just allow myself to weep. When my son arrived in our life, it crossed my mind briefly to name him after my dead brother who was in his turn named after this uncle. We did not, and I am sure this was a good decision. The transmission of unresolved grief down the generations must be interrupted somewhere. The task of proper mourning, even for those we never knew or loved directly, is a kind of responsibility.

Love revived through death

When my brother Olly died suddenly of a heart attack at the age of 58, when I was 45, a chasm opened up in me. In no sense had I been really close to him in adult life, although a deep fondness was always alive. In my childhood, he had been important in ways I had entirely forgotten. I think he was a troubled young man, with a violent edge to his nature. He was born with a bad harelip and cleft palate and spent long periods in East Grinstead hospital for surgery and reconstruction.

My parents were educated people, and my mother was highly academically motivated. But my brother did not like school and did not do well there. He left at 15 with few qualifications and became a farmhand. He owned a double-barrelled 12-bore shotgun and from time to time would shoot pigeons out of his bedroom window. All very difficult for the rector and his wife, but a source of quiet rebellious satisfaction to me and my brothers. My mother would call me in urgently and anxiously from the garden before the pastoral calm was shattered, and bloodied pigeons flapped in all directions. Olly bought ageing second-hand cars and drove them recklessly fast down country lanes. He smashed them up more than once, and by the time he married his face was noticeably scarred from these accidents, as though he needed to maim himself all over again. By now, though, so successful was all the surgery, anyone who did not know would not have guessed at his harelip. By the age of 20, I think he was probably fortunate not to have killed himself or someone else.

Olly came home to the rectory smelling of horse manure, and his bedroom reeked of sweat and dirty socks. He wrestled and roughed and tumbled with the 5- or 6-year-old me, and I loved it. He even persuaded my parents to allow me, at the age of about 8, to accompany him to see an evening's professional wrestling in some seedy venue. In the rather high-minded atmosphere of our home, he earthed me, and I came to know I had a body. Our contact was warm, visceral, and real. Neither of my parents were tactile people, and, when Olly died, it was this 5-year-old and no doubt much younger self that suddenly grieved. A deep, forgotten longing for easy, uncomplicated physical holding welled up in me. In various ways, the path of my life was suddenly disrupted, and I pitched forward in search of deeper, more connected love than I had been capable of until then. What I found takes many forms, but I often ache from the desire to fold my son in my arms. He loves to rough and tumble, but he cannot know the debt this pleasure owes to his dead uncle.

Dead babies, and alive

Olly stayed married all his life and raised three children with his wife. She also had at least one miscarriage or stillbirth (I am not quite sure which) but perhaps the event registered in my young mind partly because they did name their lost child—Lucy. The atmosphere of my remembered childhood is tinged with a kind of half-knowledge, an uncertain belief, that my mother also had two miscarriages. And this brings me to my daughter. I embarked on fatherhood later in life than most—most weeks some stranger, or child, in a playground speaks to me assuming I am their grandfather—and was very uncertain about a second child for many reasons. But for my wife it felt almost like a life-or-death decision. My own decision to embrace this choice entailed a significant rearrangement of my view of myself. I gave up thinking about "my" needs and "my" life in favour of the realization that our marriage and our family was now the primary unit of concern. I am a part of something that is bigger than the sum of its parts.

When our daughter arrived, I felt an unexpected sense of calm and completeness. My thoughts turned to my mother and the two miscarriages that are part of the story of my internal mother. It is too simple to say that I was somehow impelled to replace these lost babies of hers, because I am not certain they were ever conceived. But the psychological mother I carry inside me did have two miscarriages, and I have carried a sense of loss and inchoate grief about them. In the early weeks of my son's life, seeing me or my wife cradling him, more than one relative said, "Ah, it's all come right!" For me, holding my daughter, it was as though a dimly perceived ghost had been finally exorcized.

My father, his father, and me

So also when I was in my in my twenties, my father died after a long dementing illness. I had a lot of difficulty communicating and relating to him through this period, as did all his family, I think, and he was not a man who was ever comfortable with strong feelings or emotional pain. But one evening as I sat quietly and anxiously with him, he suddenly said to me, "I wish I could die like my father did. He sat down after lunch one day, had a heart attack and died just like that." It was the most poignant and painful communication my father ever made to me. In the midst of his suffering and disorientation, I think my grandfather's death became my father's idea of a good death. I cannot be sure, but I now suspect that my father was just appallingly lonely during these last years, exactly because no one around him could bear, or could summon the emotional resources, to find a way to come closer to him.

The sociologist Clive Seale speaks of dying people "falling from culture" (Seale, 1998) as they become more dependent and unwell in the period, sometimes lengthy, that precedes death, as they lose connection with the networks and routine relationships that are the taken-for-granted social tissue of our aliveness. Thus what he calls "social death" may often precede the death of the body. It is family and perhaps close friends who are there, or not, to accompany the dying person in his or her final period of life, and a disproportionate burden of this task falls, of course, to women. The emotional task of truly "being with" someone as they approach their death, so that they do not experience themselves as "dropped from mind" by those closest to them, is perhaps one of the greatest tests of emotional maturity that any of us will face.

I felt hopelessly inadequate in the face of my father's process of dying, and guilty for many years afterwards. Eventually it was a relief to let go of any ambivalence I felt towards him as my father and say to myself, "I wish I had been able to be a better son to you." But in writing about these memories, I came to a slightly different view of matters. His communication to me of his death wish, and my receipt of it, was not nothing. Out of the silence, the void that I remember him apparently inhabiting much of the time as he deteriorated, he *was* able to formulate this expression of his distress—in effect, of his wish to die and be released—and deliver it to me. And I was at least there to receive it. There could have been so much more, but I suspect that even such a fleeting moment of connection as this is hard won by all involved. Maybe there were other moments with my mother or other family members—I don't know. We just didn't talk properly about it. But I offer this story, and these thoughts, to provide us with some sense of the difficulties that face us as we try to think well about this idea of "relating to dying"—what we might hope for as we ourselves approach death, and what we might hope for from ourselves in relating to others in their dying. And, finally, recognizing the depth of the emotional challenge involved, the value of forgiveness for what we fail to achieve with others, or to receive from them.

This is the territory explored by Atul Gawande in his profound and important book *Being Mortal: Illness, Medicine, and What Matters in the End* (2014). In the space that lies between manic hope or denial, on the one hand, or helpless resignation in the face of the knowledge of imminent death, on the other, Gawande describes the "hard conversations" the dying and the living need to have, so that the dying can exercise maximum feasible choice about how they spend their last weeks, days and hours. Medicine has become heroically addicted to prolonging life at all costs, disabling everyone's ability to weigh the balance between longevity and quality of life in the final phases of living. "Assisted living is far harder than assisted death", writes Gawande, "but its possibilities are far greater, as well. . . . Our ultimate goal, after all, is not a good death but a good life to the very end" (2014, p. 245).

Death, dying, and the meaning of our work

If I had not already alluded to it, I am sure that by now you would have caught the drift of my narrative about myself and the biographical roots of me becoming a social worker and therapist. But do these thoughts suggest anything larger about the project of social work and social welfare? I was a post-war baby, a boomer, and a beneficiary of what have been called the "golden years" of British prosperity and social justice in which our welfare state was created and flourished. My former boss, the organizational consultant Anton Obholzer, described the unconscious social role of the NHS as being a "keep death at bay" service (Obholzer, 1994), and I believe this idea extends to social work.

It is not just that we inevitably encounter death as social workers—one of my first tasks after qualifying was to find respite care for an elderly homeless man. He settled quickly and gratefully into the home that I found as an emergency placement. But, of course, I had to move him, and a few days after the transition to his new accommodation, he died. "Your worst fear must be that you killed him by making him move", said my supervisor. She was absolutely right, and what a relief it was to hear it voiced. Child protection workers live every day in the shadow of the panicky, retributive impulses that murdered children from time to time provoke. Our society cannot yet come to terms with child torture and murder, and it turns its primitive anxiety on social workers. But beyond all this, there is more, I think.

Perhaps I am stating the obvious, but it was not physical ill-health that caused me such distress when I was forced to move home at 9 years of age, any more than it was physical ill-health that primarily "killed" my elderly client when I forced him to move homes. The terror of abandonment that lives on in the minds of so many looked-after children who have been forcibly removed from their families of origin, and then endured multiple placement changes, is not a physical illness, although it may be related to later poor physical-health outcomes. The intensity of emotional distress we encounter in young unaccompanied asylum seekers who come into our care is not primarily about their state of physical health. All these processes are what Colin Murray Parkes named "psycho-social transitions" (Parkes, 1971). Occasionally, maybe, such transitions can actually kill us, or be the last straw. Too many of them at once, or in succession, or in interaction with other vulnerability factors, is an established cause of mental ill-health, especially of depression (Brown & Harris, 1978). The poorer or more disadvantaged you are, the greater the likelihood that you will experience such debilitating losses and transitions. Loss, the mobilization of fears about dying that loss engenders, and the work of mourning that is required to negotiate such losses is the link to dying and death and the permanent undertow in our work as social workers.

When I am asked what I think social work is "really" all about, I tend to answer that it is, or should be, about the provision of skilful, supportive, psychologically attuned, and practically helpful relationships for people enduring transitions that they cannot cope with. Social welfare and health services are ultimately all about relationships, though, of course, material provision and technological kit is also essential. In societies that are grossly unequal, too poor, or simply too lacking in social compassion to provide a real safety net, people—including babies and children—die younger, and their quality of life, as well as the quality of their dying, is much worse. The US is one of the richest countries in the world and also one of the most unequal, and their health and welfare outcomes reflect the latter. Britain seems to me to be moving steadily in the same direction.

There are many stories from my life related to dying and fear of death I have not told. I had cancer—Hodgkin's Disease—twice in my twenties and stand before you today to tell the tale because I have lived in a rich country with a national health service. Singing in *Up to Me* of how death shadows us, Bob Dylan added, "At least I heard your bluebird sing". I don't know whether I've ever heard a bluebird sing, but I have had a good life. Had there been no NHS, I might still have lived, but I and my family would have been massively impoverished because the costs of private medical care would have decimated us. I spent a lot of my own money accessing psychotherapy for myself, significantly but not only to help me better manage the psychic consequences of having been so close to death so early.

We are quite privileged in this country in relation to our capacity to think, and do something, about the process of ordinary dying. The *2015 Quality of Death Index* (EIU, 2015), which ranks palliative care services globally, places the UK at the very top. And yet there is so much more to be done, and so much more to make sense of. I do not know how to make sense of living in a society that can at times take such care over dying and death, and simultaneously turn a blind eye to the catastrophes of war that now impinge upon us, most obviously in the form of "migration". Someone said recently that the unceasing war in the Middle East is now actually being conducted inside our European borders. It is not that war and populations fleeing war are "out there", while something we call "terrorism" is "in here". The war is here—and not likely to go away for a very long time.

By reflecting on my own experiences, including how wars over and done with a century ago are still emotionally alive in me, I have tried to say something about the vital humanitarian significance of this endeavour we call social work, and how it is part of what it means to live in a civilized society, and so must be defended, preserved, and if necessary fought for. This is a public project, but our private relation to death and dying must inform it. Perhaps it is presumptuous to end this chapter, and book, with an example of my own attempt to seek containment through art, but I have decided to do it. As poems sometimes do, this one more or less wrote itself, gathering together both the immediacy of an experience of the external world and a sense of my always-unresolved relation to dying and death. As in Margot Waddell's paper, "Darkness" features, as do my own children, to whom this book has been dedicated.

I sat with you awhile

Downhill my children are shadows
dancing on the ancient stone bridge.
Fractured leaves of windblown laughter
brush my skin, mingling the scent of knotted pine
that shades this seablown, seagreen
crusty seat and its weathered inscription:
Francis McLaren 1949–60.
At sea two black dinghies speed along,
distant motors whining. Other windblown lives.
I think less of him, although a pale face, baggy shorts,
and bad 1950s haircut come to mind;
more of you—bewildered, heartstoned, cleaving to the only light
not snuffed, this path and its falling away
towards a tiny rocky shore.
Here then, a place
made for others to notice that one day,
a world away, darkness fell on this whole bright land.
With this understanding (if it is true at all)
I sat with you awhile.

Note

1. King James Bible, Luke 2:49, "And he said unto them, How is it that ye sought me? Wist ye not that I must be about my Father's business?"

REFERENCES

Adlam, J., & Scanlon, C. (2005). Personality disorder and homelessness: Membership and "unhoused minds" in forensic settings. *Group Analysis, 38* (3): 452–466.

Alderdice, J., Lord (2010). Off the couch and round the conference table. In: A. Lemma & M. Patrick (Eds.), *Off the Couch: Contemporary Psychoanalytic Approaches*. Hove: Routledge.

Archer, M., Bhaskar, R., Collier, A., Lawson, T., & Norrie, A. (Eds.) (1998). *Critical Realism: Essential Readings*. London: Routledge.

Armstrong, D. (2004). Emotions in organizations: Disturbance or intelligence? In: C. Huffington, D. Armstrong. W. Halton, L. Hoyle, & J. Pooley (Eds.), *Working Below the Surface: The Emotional Life of Contemporary Organizations*. London: Karnac.

Bacon, R. (1988). Countertransference in a case conference: Resistance and rejection in work with abusing families and their children. In: G. Pearson, J. Treseder, & M. Yelloly (Eds.), *Social Work and the Legacy of Freud*. Basingstoke: Macmillan.

Bailey, H. (2015). "I want my social worker". One child's struggle to find an available maternal figure: Reflections from a peer supervision group. *Journal of Social Work Practice, 29* (2): 223–229.

Barlow, J., & Scott, J. (2010). *Safeguarding in the 21st Century—Where to Now?* Totnes: Research in Practice.

Bateman, A., & Fonagy, P. (2006). *Mentalization-based Treatment for Borderline Personality Disorder*. Oxford: Oxford University Press.

Bauman, Z. (1992). *Mortality, Immortality and Other Life Strategies*. Cambridge: Polity Press.

Beckett, C. (2003). The language of siege: Military metaphors in the spoken language of social work. *British Journal of Social Work, 33* (5): 625–639.

Bion, W. R. (1962). *Learning from Experience*. London: Karnac.

Bion, W. R. (1970). *Attention and Interpretation. A Scientific Approach to Insight in Psycho-Analysis and Groups*. London: Tavistock Publications. Reprinted London: Karnac, 1984.

Bion, W. R. (1990). *Brazilian Lectures: 1973, São Paulo; 1974, Rio de Janeiro/São Paulo*. London: Karnac.

Bion, W. R. (1994). Evidence. In: *Clinical Seminars and Other Works* (pp. 313–320). London: Karnac.

Blaikie, N. (1993). *Approaches to Social Enquiry*. Cambridge: Polity Press.

Bollas, C. (1987). *The Shadow of the Object: Psychoanalysis of the Unthought Known*. London: Free Association Books.

Bourdieu, P. (1999). *The Weight of the World*. Cambridge: Polity Press.

Bower, M. (2005a). Psychoanalytic theories for social work practice. In: M. Bower (Ed.), *Psychoanalytic Theory for Social Work Practice: Thinking under Fire* (pp. 3–14). Abingdon: Routledge.

Bower, M. (Ed.) (2005b). *Psychoanalytic Theory for Social Work Practice: Thinking under Fire*. Abingdon: Routledge.

Bower, M., & Solomon, R. (2017). *What Social Workers Need to Know: A Psychoanalytic Approach*. London: Routledge.

BPC (2008a). *British Psychoanalytic Council Newsletter*, October.

BPC (2008b). *Position Statement on Statutory Regulation and Other Issues*. London: British Psychoanalytic Council.

Brandon, M., Sidebotham, P., Bailey, S., Belderson, P., Hawley, C., Ellis, C., & Megson, M. (2012). *New Learning from Serious Case Reviews: A Two Year Report for 2009–2011*. London: Department for Education.

Briggs, S. (1997). *Growth and Risk in Infancy*. London: Jessica Kingsley.

Britton, R. (1989). The missing link: Parental sexuality in the Oedipus complex. In: R. Britton, M. Feldman, & E. O'Shaughnessy, *The Oedipus Complex. Today: Clinical Implications* (pp. 83–101). London: Karnac.

Britton, R. (1998). Before and after the depressive position: Ps(n)→D(n)→ Ps(n+1). In: *Belief and Imagination* (pp. 69–81). London: Routledge.

Broadhurst, K., Wastell, D., White, S., Hall, C., Peckover, S., Thompson, K., et al. (2010). Performing "Initial Assessment": Identifying the latent conditions for error at the front-door of local authority children's services. *British Journal of Social Work, 40* (2): 352–370.

Brown, G., & Harris, T. (1978). *Social Origins of Depression*. London: Tavistock.

Brown, J. (2006). Reflexivity in the research process: Psychoanalytic observations. *International Journal of Social Research Methodology: Theory and Practice, 9* (3): 181–197.

Burton, S. (2009). *The Oversight and Review of Cases in the Light of Changing Circumstances and New Information: How Do People Respond to New (and Challenging) Information?* London: C4EO.

Byrne, D. (1998). *Complexity Theory and the Social Sciences*. London: Routledge.

Casement, P. (1985). Forms of interactive communication. In: *On Learning from the Patient* (pp. 72–101). Hove: Routledge.

Chapman, J. (2004). *System Failure: Why Governments Must Learn to Think Differently* (2nd edition). London: Demos.

Chasseguet-Smirgel, J. (1985). *Creativity and Perversion*. London: Free Association Books.

Clarke, S., & Hoggett, P. (Eds.) (2009). *Researching beneath the Surface: Psycho-Social Research Methods in Practice*. London: Karnac.

Coleman, W. (2006). The analytic super-ego. *Journal of the British Association of Psychotherapists, 44* (2): 99–114.

Cooper, A. (1996). Psychoanalysis and the politics of organisational theory. *Journal of Social Work Practice, 10* (2): 137–145.

Cooper, A. (1997). Thinking the unthinkable: "White liberal" defences against understanding in anti-racist training. *Journal of Social Work Practice, 11* (2): 127–137.

Cooper, A. (2005a). Surface and depth in the Victoria Climbié report. *Child and Family Social Work, 10*: 1–9.

Cooper, A. (2005b). Surface and depth in the Victoria Climbié inquiry report: Exploring emotionally intelligent policy. In: A. Cooper & J. Lousada, *Borderline Welfare: Feeling and Fear of Feeling in Modern Welfare* (pp. 145–169). London: Karnac.

Cooper, A. (2008a). *Gods, Devils and Murderers: Health and Welfare in a Secular Age*. Unpublished paper given at the Annual Regional Study Day for Medical Practitioners, Tampere, Finland.

Cooper, A. (2008b). Misguided vengeance. *The Guardian*, 2 December. Available at: https://www.theguardian.com/commentisfree/2008/dec/02/baby-p-haringey-social-services-sackings

Cooper, A. (2008c). Welfare: Dead, dying or just transubstantiated? *Soundings, 38*.

Cooper, A. (2009). "Be quiet and listen": Emotion, public policy and social totality. In: S. Day Sclater, D. W. Jones, H. Price, & C. Yates (Eds.), *Emotion: New Psychosocial Perspectives* (pp. 169–182). London: Routledge.

Cooper, A. (2010). Legend, myth and idea: On the fate of a great paper. *British Journal of Psychotherapy, 26* (2): 219–227.

Cooper, A. (2011). How to (almost) murder a profession: The unsolved mystery of British social work. In: J. Adlam, A. Aiyegbusi, P. Kleinot, A. Motz, & C. Scanlon (Eds.), *The Therapeutic Milieu under Fire* (pp. 145–161). London: Jessica Kingsley.

Cooper, A. (2014). A short psychosocial history of British child abuse and protection: Case studies of problems of mourning in the public sphere. *Journal of Social Work Practice, 28* (3): 271–285.

Cooper, A., & Dartington, T. (2004). The vanishing organization: Organizational containment in a networked world. In: C. Huffington, D. Armstrong, W. Halton, L. Hoyle, & J. Pooley (Eds.), *Working Below the Surface: The Emotional Life of Contemporary Organizations* (pp. 127–150). London: Karnac.

Cooper, A., & Lees, A. (2014). Spotlit: Defences against anxiety in contemporary human service organizations. In: D. Armstrong & M. Rustin (Eds.), *Social Defences against Anxiety: Explorations in the Paradigm* (pp. 239–255). London: Karnac.

Cooper, A., & Lousada, J. (2005). *Borderline Welfare: Fear and Fear of Feeling in Modern Welfare.* London: Karnac.

Cooper, A., & Whittaker, A. (2014). History as tragedy, never as farce: Tracing the long cultural narrative of child protection in England. *Journal of Social Work Practice, 28* (3): 251–266.

Costall, A. (2010). The future of experimental psychology. *The Psychologist, 23* (12): 1022–1223.

Craig, P., Dieppe, P., Macintyre, S., Michie, S., Nazareth, I., & Petticrew, M. (2008). *Developing and Evaluating Complex Interventions: New Guidance.* London: Medical Research Council. Available at: www.mrc.ac.uk/complexinterventionsguidance

Cusk, R. (2002). *A Life's Work: On Becoming a Mother*. London: Fourth Estate.

Dalal, F. (2008). Against the celebration of diversity. *British Journal of Psychotherapy, 24* (1): 4–19.

Dartington, T. (2010). *Managing Vulnerability: The Underlying Dynamics of Systems of Care.* London: Karnac.

Daston, L., & Galison, P. (2007). *Objectivity*. Brooklyn, NY: Zone Books.

Davids, F. (2003). The internal racist. *Bulletin of the British Psychoanalytical Society, 39* (4): 1–15.

Davies, W. (2015). *The Happiness Industry: How the Government and Big Business Sold Us Well-Being.* London: Verso.

Deacon, J. (2010). *From Perversion to Policy.* Doctoral thesis, University of East London and the Tavistock and Portman NHS Trust, London.

Derrida, J. (1988). *Limited Inc.* Evanston, IL: Northwestern University Press.

DfES (2003). *Every Child Matters.* Norwich: TSO. Available at: https://www.gov.uk/government/uploads/system/uploads/attachment_data/file/272064/5860.pdf

Eagleton, T. (2009). *Reason, Faith and Revolution: Reflections on the God Debate.* Princeton, NJ: Yale University Press.

Eissold, K. (1994). The intolerance of diversity in psychoanalytic institutes. *International Journal of Psychoanalysis, 75*: 785–800.

EIU (2015). *The 2015 Quality of Death Index: Ranking Palliative Care Across the World.* London: The Economist Intelligence Unit. Available at: https://www.eiuperspectives.economist.com/sites/default/files/2015%20EIU%20Quality%20of%20Death%20Index%20Oct%2029%20FINAL.pdf

Eliot, G. (1871). *Middlemarch.* London: Blackwood.

Eliot, T. S. (1962). *T.S. Eliot: The Complete Poems and Plays 1909–1950.* New York: Harcourt, Brace & World.

Etzioni, A. (1967). Mixed scanning: A "third" approach to decision making. *Public Administration Review, 27*: 385–392.

Evans, J. (2003). Vigilance and vigilantes: Thinking psychoanalytically about anti-paedophile action. *Theoretical Criminology, 7* (2): 163–189.

Ferguson, H. (2005). Working with violence, the emotions and the psychosocial dynamics of child protection: Reflections on the Victoria Climbié case. *Social Work Education, 24* (7): 781–795.

Feyerabend, P. (1975). *Against Method.* London: Verso.

Foster, J. (2009). *Thinking on the Front Line: Why Some Social Work Teams Struggle and Others Thrive.* Doctoral thesis, University of East London and the Tavistock and Portman NHS Trust, London.

Foster, J. (2016). *Building Effective Social Work Teams.* Abingdon: Routledge.

Fraiberg, S., Adelson, E., & Shapiro, V. (1975). Ghosts in the nursery: A psychoanalytic approach to the problems of impaired mother–infant relationships. *Journal of the American Academy of Child Psychiatry, 14* (3): 387–421.

Freedland, J. (2015). Labour must learn to speak human, whatever its policies. *The Guardian*, 17 July.

Freire, P. (1996). *Pedagogy of the Oppressed* (revised edition). New York: Continuum.

Freud, S. (1905e). Fragment of an analysis of a case of hysteria [Dora]. *Case Histories I.* London: Penguin, 1977.

Freud, S. (1915e). The unconscious. *Standard Edition, 14.*

Freud, S. (1916–17). *Introductory Lectures on Psycho-Analysis, Standard Edition, 16.*

Freud, S. (1917e). Mourning and melancholia. *Standard Edition, 14.*

Freud, S. (1918b). From the history of an infantile neurosis. *Standard Edition, 17.*

Freud, S. (1919a). Lines of advance in psycho-analytic therapy. *Standard Edition, 17.*

Freud, S. (1930a). *Civilization and Its Discontents. Standard Edition, 21.*

Gawande, A. (2014). *Being Mortal: Illness, Medicine, and What Matters in the End.* London: Profile Books.

Gibbs, R. (2013). *Standing in the Shadows: Faith, Homelessness and Troubled Lives.* Doctoral dissertation, University of East London, London.

Giddens, A. (1979). *Central Problems of Social Theory.* London: Macmillan.

Giddens, A. (1984). *The Constitution of Society.* Cambridge: Polity Press.

Gilbert, R., Spatz Widom, C., Browne, K., Fergusson, D., Webb, E., & Janson, S. (2008). Burden and consequences of child maltreatment in high-income countries. *The Lancet, 373* (9657): 68–81. Available at: www.thelancet.com/journals/lancet/article/PIIS0140-6736(08)61706-7/fulltext

Gilligan, J. (1996). *Violence: Reflections on Our Deadliest Epidemic.* London: Jessica Kingsley.

Glaser, B. G., & Strauss, A. L. (2009). *The Discovery of Grounded Theory: Strategies for Qualitative Research.* New Brunswick, NJ: Transaction Publishers.

Goodman, S., Trowler, I., & Munro, E. (2011). *Social Work Reclaimed: Innovative Frameworks for Child and Family Social Work Practice.* London: Jessica Kingsley.

Goretti, G. R. (2007). Projective identification: A theoretical investigation of the concept starting from "Notes on Some Schizoid Mechanisms". *International Journal of Psychoanalysis, 88* (2): 387–405.

Gross, K. (2015). *Late Fragments: Everything I Want to Tell You (About This Magnificent Life).* London: HarperCollins.

Halton, W. (2014). Obsessional punitive defences in care systems: Menzies Lyth revisited. In: D. Armstrong & M. Rustin (Eds.), *Social Defences against Anxiety: Explorations in a Paradigm* (pp. 27–38). London: Karnac.

Hammersley, M. (1992). *What's Wrong with Ethnography?* London: Routledge.

Hard, E., Rock, J., & Stern, J. (2015). Paradigms, politics and pragmatics: Psychotherapy in primary care in City and Hackney—A new model for the NHS. Part 2: Operational model, practice and outcomes. *Psychoanalytic Psychotherapy, 29* (2): 139–159.

HBO (2006). Soft eyes. *The Wire*, Season 4, Episode 2 [DVD]. New York: Home Box Office.

HBO (2008). *The Wire: The Complete 5th Season* [DVD]. New York: Home Box Office.

Healy, K. (1998). Clinical audit and conflict. In: R. Davenhill & M. Patrick (Eds.), *Rethinking Clinical Audit: The Case of Psychotherapy Services in the NHS* (pp. 38–56). London: Routledge.

Hingley-Jones, H. (2008). *"Trying Transitions": Researching the Identity Development of Severely Learning Disabled Adolescents. A Psychosocial, Observational Study*. Doctoral thesis, University of East London and the Tavistock and Portman NHS Trust, London.

Hingley-Jones, H., & Ruch, G. (2016). "Stumbling through"? Relationship-based social work practice in austere times. *Journal of Social Work Practice, 30* (3): 235–248.

Hinshelwood, R. D., & Skogstad, W. (Eds.) (2000). *Observing Organisations: Anxiety, Defence and Culture in Health Care*. London: Routledge.

Hirschhorn, L. (1997). *Reworking Authority: Leading and Following in the Post-Modern Age*. Cambridge, MA: MIT Press.

HMSO (1988). *Report of the Inquiry into Child Abuse in Cleveland 1987*. London: Her Majesty's Stationery Office.

Hoffmeyer, J. (1996). *Signs of Meaning in the Universe*. Bloomington, IN: Indiana University Press.

Hoggett, P. (2008). What's in a hyphen? Reconstructing psychosocial studies. *Psychoanalysis, Culture & Society, 13*: 379–384.

Hoggett, P. (2010). Government and the perverse social defence. *British Journal of Psychotherapy, 26* (2): 202–212.

Hoggett, P. (2014). Learning from three practices. *Journal of Psycho-Social Studies, 8* (1).

Hollway, W. (2015). *Knowing Mothers: Researching Maternal Identity Change*. Basingstoke: Palgrave Macmillan.

Hollway, W., & Jefferson, T. (2012). *Doing Qualitative Research Differently: A Psychosocial Approach*. London: Sage.

Holmes, J. (2002). Narcissism. In: I. Ward (Ed.), *On a Darkling Plain: Journeys into the Unconscious* (pp. 173–203). Cambridge: Icon Books.

Hutten, J., Bazalgette, J., & Armstrong, D. (1994). What does management really mean? In: R. Casemore, G. Dyos, A. Eden, K. Kellner, J. McAuley, & S. Moss (Eds.), *What Makes Consultancy Work: Understanding the Dynamics* (pp. 185–203). London: South Bank University Press.

Hutton, W. (1996). *The State We're In*. London: Vintage.

Ingham, G., & Fitzgerald, G. (1988). An introduction to the inter-cultural psychotherapy seminars. *Journal of Social Work Practice, 3* (3): 1–7.

Jordan, S. (2015). *That Joke Isn't Funny Anymore: Humour, Jokes and Their Relationship to Social Work.* Doctoral thesis, University of East London and the Tavistock and Portman NHS Trust, London.

Keats, J. (1817). Letter to George and Thomas Keats, 21st December. In: *The Letters of John Keats: A Selection*, ed. R. Gittings. Oxford: Oxford University Press, 1970.

Khan, M. (1986). The concept of cumulative trauma. In: G. Kohon (Ed.), *The British School of Psychoanalysis: The Independent Tradition* (pp. 117–135). London: Free Association Books.

Klein, M. (1940). Mourning and its relation to manic-depressive states. In: *Love, Guilt and Reparation* (pp. 344–369). London: Hogarth Press, 1975.

Kraemer, S. (2009). Is there another word for it? Countertransference in family therapy. In: C. Flaskas & D. Pocock (Eds.), *Systems and Psychoanalysis: Contemporary Integrations in Family Therapy* (pp. 39–56). London: Karnac.

Kraemer, S. (2011). "The dangers of this atmosphere": A Quaker connection in the Tavistock Clinic's development. *History of the Human Sciences, 24* (2): 82–102.

Krantz, J. (2010). Social defences and twenty-first century organizations. *British Journal of Psychotherapy, 26* (2): 192–201.

Kuhn, T. S. (1975). *The Structure of Scientific Revolutions* (2nd edition, enlarged). Chicago, IL: University of Chicago Press.

La Fontaine, J. (1994). *The Extent and Nature of Organised and Ritual Abuse: Research Findings*. London: HMSO.

Laming, Lord W. H. (2003). *The Victoria Climbié Inquiry: Report*. Norwich: TSO. Available at: https://www.gov.uk/government/uploads/system/uploads/attachment_data/file/273183/5730.pdf

Lanchester, J. (2010). *Whoops! Why Everyone Owes Everyone and No One Can Pay*. London: Penguin, Allen Lane.

Leader, D. (2009). *The New Black: Mourning, Melancholia and Depression.* London: Penguin.

Lees, A. (2014). *Spotlights and Shadows: A Social Work Perspective on Information Sharing to Safeguard Children.* Doctoral thesis, University of Southampton.

Lees, A., Meyer, E., & Rafferty, J. (2011). From Menzies Lyth to Munro: The problem of managerialism. *British Journal of Social Work, 43* (3): 542–558.

Lieberson, S. (1997). The big broad issues in society and social history: Application of a probabilistic perspective. In: V. R. McKim & S. P. Turner (Eds.), *Causality in Crisis? Statistical Methods and the Search for Causal Knowledge in the Social Sciences* (pp. 359–385). Notre Dame, IN: University of Notre Dame Press.

Lindblom, C. (1959). The science of muddling through. *Public Administration Review, 19*: 78–88.

Liotti, G., Mollon, P., & Miti, G. (2007). Dissociative disorders. In G. Gabbard, S. Beck, & G. Holmes (Eds.), *Oxford Textbook of Psychotherapy* (pp. 203–211). Oxford: Oxford University Press.

Lowe, F. (Ed.) (2014). *Thinking Space: Promoting Thinking about Race, Culture, and Diversity in Psychotherapy and Beyond*. London: Karnac.

Mandin, P. (2014). *Creating a Space to Think in a Structured World: An Exploration of the Structures, Relationships and Emotions Emerging in Network Meetings in the Wider Context of Child Care Proceedings*. Doctoral thesis, University of East London and the Tavistock and Portman NHS Trust, London.

Mattinson, J., Sinclair, I., Coussell, P., & Morley, R. (1979). *Mate and Stalemate: Working with Marital Problems in a Social Services Department*. London: Basil Blackwell.

Menzies, I. E. P. (1959). A case study in the functioning of social systems as a defence against anxiety: A report on a study of the nursing service of a general hospital. *Human Relations, 13* (1960): 95–121. Reprinted in I. Menzies Lyth, *Containing Anxiety in Institutions*. London: Free Association Books, 1988.

Miller, A. (1958). *Death of a Salesman*. In: *Collected Plays: Arthur Miller*. London: Cresset Press.

Mitchell, S. D. (2009). *Unsimple Truths: Science, Complexity and Policy*. Chicago, IL: University of Chicago Press.

Mollon, P. (2002). *Remembering Trauma: A Psychotherapists Guide to Memory and Illusion* (2nd edition). London: Whurr.

Munro, E. (2010). *The Munro Review of Child Protection. Part One—A Systems Analysis*. London: The Stationery Office. Available at: https://www.gov.uk/government/publications/munro-review-of-child-protection-final-report-a-child-centred-system

Munro, E. (2011a). *The Munro Review of Child Protection: Interim Report—The Child's Journey*. London: The Stationery Office. Available at: https://www.gov.uk/government/publications/munro-review-of-child-protection-final-report-a-child-centred-system

Munro, E. (2011b). *The Munro Review of Child Protection: Final Report—A Child-Centred System*. London: The Stationery Office. Available at: https://www.gov.uk/government/publications/munro-review-of-child-protection-final-report-a-child-centred-system

Noyes, C. (2015). *Live Work: Creativity on the Front Line*. Doctoral thesis, University of East London and the Tavistock and Portman NHS Trust, London.

Obholzer, A. (1989). Psychoanalysis and the political process. *Psychoanalytic Psychotherapy, 4* (1): 55–66.

Obholzer, A. (1994). Managing social anxieties in public sector organizations. In: A. Obholzer & V. Zagier Roberts (Eds.), *The Unconscious at Work: Individual and Organizational Stress in the Human Services* (pp. 169–178). London: Routledge.

Obholzer, A., & Zagier Roberts, V. (Eds.) (1994). *The Unconscious at Work: Individual and Organizational Stress in the Human Services*. London: Routledge.

Ogden, T. H. (1999). *Reverie and Interpretation: Sensing Something Human*. London: Karnac.

O'Sullivan, N. (2017). *The Dichotomy of Thinking and Doing*. Doctoral thesis, University of East London and the Tavistock and Portman NHS Trust, London.

Parkes, C. M. (1971). Psycho-social transitions: A field for study. *Social Science & Medicine (1967), 5* (2): 101–115.

Parton, N. (2008). Changes in the form of knowledge in social work: From the "social" to the "informational"? *British Journal of Social Work, 38* (2): 253–269.

Pawson, R. (2006). *Evidence-based Policy: A Realist Perspective*. London: Sage.

Pawson, R., & Tilley, N. (1997). *Realistic Evaluation*. London: Sage.

Potamianou, A. (1997). *Hope: A Shield in the Economy of Borderline States*. London: Routledge.

Power, M. (1994). *The Audit Explosion*. London: Demos.

Preston-Shoot, M., & Agass, D. (1990). *Making Sense of Social Work: Psychodynamics, Systems and Practice*. London: Macmillan.

Price, H. (2004). *The Emotional Context of Young Children's Literacy Learning*. Doctoral thesis, University of East London, London.

Price, H., & Cooper, A. (2012). In the field: Psychoanalytic observation and epistemological realism. In: C. Urwin & J. Sternberg (Eds.), *Infant Observation and Research: Emotional Processes in Everyday Lives* (pp. 55–65). Hove: Routledge.

Price, H., Herd, J., Jones, D., & Sampson, A. (2017). *A Qualitative Evaluation of the Mulberry Bush School*. London: University of East London.

Pritchard, C., & Williams, R. (2010). Comparing possible "child-abuse-related-deaths" in England and Wales with the major developed countries in 1974–2006: Signs of progress? *British Journal of Social Work, 40* (6): 1710–1718.

Ragin, C. (2008). *Redesigning Social Inquiry: Fuzzy Sets and Beyond*. Chicago, IL: University of Chicago Press.

Reder, P., & Duncan, S. (2004). From Colwell to Climbié: Inquiring into fatal child abuse. In: N. Stanley & J. Manthorpe (Eds.), *The Age of the Inquiry: Learning and Blaming in Health and Social Care* (pp. 92–115). London: Routledge.

Richards, B. (2007). *Emotional Governance: Politics, Media, Terror*. Basingstoke: Palgrave Macmillan.

Richards, B. (2018). *What Holds Us Together?* London: Karnac.

Rickman, J. (2003). A study of Quaker beliefs. In: P. King (Ed.), *No Ordinary Psychoanalyst: The Exceptional Contributions of John Rickman* (pp. 269–293). London: Karnac.

Rubenfeld, J. (2007). *The Interpretation of Murder*. New York: Henry Holt.

Ruch, G., Turney, D., & Ward, A. (2010). *Relationship-based Practice: Getting to the Heart of Practice*. London: Jessica Kingsley.

Russell, K. (2015). *Psychosocial Concerns and Individual Anxieties for Fathers with Testicular Cancer*. Doctoral thesis, University of East London and the Tavistock and Portman NHS Trust, London.

Rustin, M. E. (2005). Conceptual analysis of critical moments in Victoria Climbié's life. *Child & Family Social Work, 10* (1): 11–19.

Rustin, M. E. (2008). Work discussion: Some historical and theoretical observations. In: M. Rustin & J. Bradley (Eds.), *Work Discussion: Learning from Reflective Practice with Children and Families* (pp. 3–21). London: Karnac.

Rustin, M., & Bradley, J. (Eds.) (2008). *Work Discussion: Learning from Reflective Practice in Work with Children and Families*. London: Karnac.

Rustin, M. J. (1991a). *The Good Society and the Inner World*. London: Verso.

Rustin, M. J. (1991b). The social organisation of secrets. In: *The Good Society and the Inner World* (pp. 87–113). London: Verso.

Rustin, M. J. (1995). Lacan, Klein and politics. In: A. Elliot & S. Frosh (Eds.), *Psychoanalysis in Contexts* (pp. 223–245). London: Routledge.

Rustin, M. J. (1997). What do we see in the nursery? Infant observation as "laboratory work". *Infant Observation, 1* (1): 93–110.

Rustin, M. J. (2006). Infant observation research: What have we learned so far? *Infant Observation, 9* (1): 35–52.

Salzberger-Wittenberg, I. (1970). *Psychoanalytic Insight and Relationships: A Kleinian Approach*. London: Routledge.

Seale, C. (1998). *Constructing Death: The Sociology of Dying and Bereavement*. Cambridge: Cambridge University Press.

Searles, H. F. (1975). Countertransference and theoretical model. In: J. G. Gunderson & L. R. Mosher (Eds.), *Psychotherapy of Schizophrenia* (pp. 223–228). New York: Jason Aronson.

Shoesmith, S. (2016). *Learning from Baby P: The Politics of Blame, Fear and Denial*. London: Jessica Kingsley.

Showalter, E. (1997). *Hystories: Hysterical Epidemics and Modern Culture.* London: Picador.

Skogstad, W. (2004). Psychoanalytic observation: The mind as research instrument. *Organisational and Social Dynamics, 4* (1): 67–87.

Smith, S. (2007). Projective processes on the front line. *Journal of Social Work Practice, 21* (2): 207–218.

Srivastava, R. (2016). How do people die from cancer? *The Guardian*, 17 August. Available at: http://www.theguardian.com/commentisfree/2016/aug/17/how-do-people-die-from-cancer-google?CMP=Share_AndroidApp_Gmail

Steiner, J. (2006). Seeing and being seen: Narcissistic pride and narcissistic humiliation. *International Journal of Psychoanalysis, 87*: 939–951.

Stevens, I., & Cox, P. (2008). Complexity theory: Developing new understandings of child protection and in residential care. *British Journal of Social Work, 338* (7): 1320–1336.

Strauss, A., & Corbin, J. (1998). *Basics of Qualitative Research: Techniques and Procedures for Developing Grounded Theory*. Thousand Oaks, CA: Sage.

Tansella, M., & Thornicroft, G. (2009). Implementation science: Understanding the translation of evidence into practice. *British Journal of Psychiatry, 195*: 283–285.

Taylor, D. (2007). *What Immortal Hand or Eye?* Paper presented at a Tavistock Clinic Scientific Meeting, London.

Taylor, H. (2013). *UK Psychoanalysis: Mistaking the Part for the Whole.* British Psychoanalytic Council Discussion Paper.

Taylor, H., Beckett, C., & McKeigue, B. (2008). Judgements of Solomon: Anxieties and defences of social workers involved in care proceedings. *Child and Family Social Work, 13*: 23–31.

Thorpe, C. (2007). Introduction. In: C. Thorpe & J. Trowell (Eds.), *Re-Rooted Lives: Interdisciplinary Work within the Family Justice System* (pp. xiii–xvi). Bristol: Jordan Publishing.

Toasland, J. (2007). Containing the container: An exploration of the containing role of management in a social work context. *Journal of Social Work Practice, 21* (2): 197–202.

Trevithick, P. (2011). Understanding defences and defensiveness in social work. *Journal of Social Work Practice, 25* (4): 389–412.

Trowell, J. (1997). Discussion. In: J. Sandler & P. Fonagy (Eds.), *Recovered Memories of Abuse: True or False?* (pp. 22–25). London: Karnac.

Tydeman, B. (2007). What is "True enough" to be convincing evidence? The child psychotherapist, the family, the team and the court. In: C. Thorpe & J. Trowell (Eds.), *Re-Rooted Lives: Interdisciplinary Work within the Family Justice System* (pp. 29–38). Bristol: Jordan Publishing.

Urwin, C., & Sternberg, J. (Eds.) (2012). *Infant Observation and Research: Emotional Processes in Everyday Life*. Hove: Routledge.

Volkan, V. (2008). *Large Group Identity, International Relations and Psychoanalysis*. Paper given at the Deutsche Psychoanalytische Gesellschaft e.V. (DGP) Meeting, Gasteig Cultural Center, Rosenheimer Platz, 23 May.

Wall, Lord Justice (2007). Child sexual abuse hearings in family courts: The role of judges and the value of expert witnesses. In: C. Thorpe & J. Trowell (Eds.), *Re-Rooted Lives: Interdisciplinary Work within the Family Justice System* (pp. 13–23). Bristol: Jordan Publishing.

Waterhouse, L., & McGhee, J. (2009). Anxiety and child protection—implications for practitioner–parent relations. *Child & Family Social Work, 14* (4): 481–490.

Weintrobe, S. (Ed.) (2013). *Engaging with Climate Change: Psychoanalytic and Interdisciplinary Perspectives*. London: Routledge.

Weiskrantz, L. (1997). Memories of abuse or abuse of memories? In J. Sandler & P. Fonagy (Eds.), *Recovered Memories of Abuse: True or False?* (pp. 3–21). London: Karnac.

Whittaker, A. (2011). Social defences and organisational culture in a local authority child protection setting: Challenges for the Munro Review? *Journal of Social Work Practice, 25* (4): 481–495.

Wilkinson, R., & Pickett, K. (2009). *The Spirit Level: Why More Equal Societies Almost Always Do Better*. London: Allen Lane.

Williams, P. (2002). The competent boundary spanner. *Public Administration, 80* (1): 103–124.

Williams, R. (1993). *Drama from Ibsen to Brecht*. London: Hogarth Press.

Wilson, K., Ruch, G., Lymbery, M., & Cooper, A. (2008). Modern social work in context: Policy, politics and organisations. In: *Social Work: An Introduction to Contemporary Practice* (pp. 28–46). London: Pearson Education.

Wilson, K., Ruch, G., Lymbery, M., & Cooper, A. (2011). *Social Work: An Introduction to Contemporary Practice* (2nd edition). London: Pearson Education.

Winnicott, D. W. (1965). The mentally ill in your caseload. In: *The Maturational Processes and the Facilitating Environment: Studies in the Theory of Emotional Development* (pp. 217–229). London: Hogarth Press.

Winnicott, D. W. (1971a). The place where we live. In: *Playing and Reality* (pp. 104–110). London: Tavistock Publications; reprinted London: Routledge, 1991.

Winnicott, D. W. (1971b). *Playing and Reality*. London: Tavistock Publications; reprinted London: Routledge, 1991.

Wittgenstein, L. (1974). *Tractatus Logico-Philosophicus*. London: Routledge & Kegan Paul.

Wood, M., & Hollis, F. (1990). *Casework: A Psychosocial Therapy*. New York: McGraw-Hill.

Woodhouse, D., & Pengelly, P. (1992). *Anxiety and the Dynamics of Collaboration*. Aberdeen: Aberdeen University Press.

Woods, D. D., Dekker, S., Cook, R., Johannesen, L., & Sarter, N. (2010). *Behind Human Error* (2nd edition). Farnham: Ashgate.

Wright Mills, C. (1959). *The Sociological Imagination*. London: Oxford University Press, 1970.

INDEX